Two-Dimensional and M-Mode Echocardiography for the Small Animal Practitioner

T0176745

The *Rapid Reference* Series

Books in the *Rapid Reference* series are ideal quick references, using a concise, practical approach to provide small animal practitioners with fast access to essential information. Designed to be used at a patient's side, these books make it easy to quickly diagnose and treat patients. With a spiral binding to lie flat, *Rapid Reference* books are an indispensable tool for the exam room.

Other *Rapid Reference Series* Titles

Life-Threatening Cardiac Emergencies for the Small Animal Practitioner
By Maureen McMichael and Ryan Fries

Two-Dimensional and M-Mode Echocardiography for the Small Animal Practitioner

SECOND EDITION

June A. Boon MS

Instructor and Echocardiographer
College of Veterinary Medicine and Biomedical Sciences
Colorado State University
Fort Collins, Colorado, USA

WILEY Blackwell

Library of Congress Cataloging-in-Publication Data

Names: Boon, June A., author.
Title: Two-dimensional and M-mode echocardiography for the small animal practitioner / June A. Boon.
Description: Second edition. | Ames, Iowa : John Wiley & Sons Inc., 2017. | Includes bibliographical references and index.
Identifiers: LCCN 2017015710| ISBN 9781119028536 (pbk.) | ISBN 9781119028550 (Adobe PDF) | ISBN 9781119028567 (epub)
Subjects: LCSH: Veterinary echocardiography. | MESH: Echocardiography–veterinary | Handbooks
Classification: LCC SF811 .B663 2017 | NLM SF 811 | DDC 636.089/61207543–dc23
LC record available at https://lccn.loc.gov/2017015710

A catalogue record for this book is available from the British Library.

SKY10078549_062824

This book is dedicated to my family – you all make my life rich.

Contents

Preface

With increasing affordability, ultrasound equipment has made its way into many private practices. Whilst entire books and sections of large books are devoted to the study of cardiac ultrasound, this handbook is meant to be a starter resource and a quick handy reference for fundamental echocardiographic information, and is by no means a comprehensive resource on veterinary echocardiography. The handbook starts with the controls on your machine, because presets do not always work well, moves on to discussing normal imaging planes and their sub-jective assessment, discusses how to obtain the imaging planes, then covers basic measurements of size and function, and finally reviews the typical features of common acquired heart disease. Videos of technique and features of disease are utilized to help you develop the skill necessary to perform the echocardiogram and aid in its interpretation. As with any skill set, it will require practice, patience and more in-depth reading to develop these techniques and assessments.

About the Companion Website

This book is accompanied by a companion website:

www.wiley.com/go/boon/two-dimensional

The website includes:
- Supplementary videos clips that demonstrate scanning techniques and disease features.
- A play icon ⊳ appears in the margin whenever a relevant video clip is available on the website.
- Each video corresponds to certain figures within the text, appearing beside the video for ease of reference.
- The password for the site is the last word in the caption for Figure 3.10.

Chapter 1 The Basics

Echocardiographic Applications

- Evaluation of:
  - Valve morphology
  - Chamber sizes
  - Wall thickness
  - Myocardial function
  - Pericardial effusion
- Aid in the Diagnosis of:
  - Chronic valve disease
  - Endocarditis
  - Cardiomyopathies (hypertrophic, dilated, unclassified)
  - Pericardial effusions
  - Cardiac neoplasia
  - Pulmonary hypertension
  - Congenital heart disease

Two-Dimensional and M-Mode Echocardiography for the Small Animal Practitioner, Second Edition. June A. Boon.
© 2017 John Wiley & Sons, Inc. Published 2017 by John Wiley & Sons, Inc.
Companion Website: www.wiley.com/go/boon/two-dimensional

Some Indications for an Echocardiogram

- Coughing
- Exercise intolerance
- Arrhythmia
- Pulmonary edema
- Pulmonary congestion
- Collapse or syncope
- Murmurs
- Cyanosis
- Lethargy
- Weak pulses
- Radiographic evidence of heart enlargement

Cardiac Anatomy

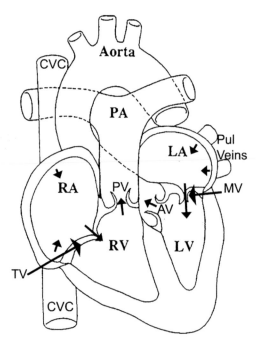

Figure 1.1 Heart Diagram. Diagram of the heart showing the chambers, valves and vessels of the heart. Flow through the heart is indicated. Note the relationships between the mitral valve and the aorta, and the pulmonary artery and the tricuspid valve. For details of abbreviations used in the figures, see the Glossary.

Orientation of the Heart in the Thorax

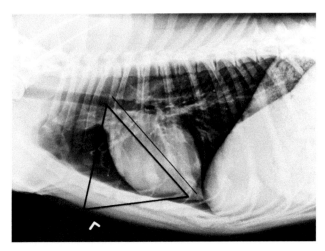

Figure 1.2 Canine lateral thoracic radiograph. This lateral radiograph shows the typical orientation of the dog's heart in the thorax. The triangle superimposed over this radiograph represents the sheet of sound coming from the transducer. Note that the transducer crystals need to be directed to the mid lumbar spine in order to create the long-axis image. Short-axis echocardiographic images of the heart have the sheet of sound oriented 90° to the long axis.

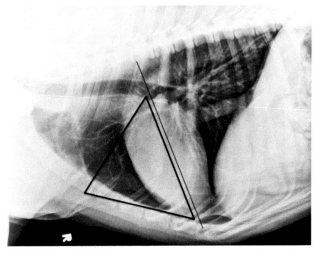

Figure 1.3 Canine lateral thoracic radiograph – deep-chested dog. This lateral radiograph shows the typical orientation of the dog's heart in the thorax when the dog has a deep chest, such as the Doberman Pinscher, Irish Wolfhound and the German Shepherd. The triangle superimposed over this radiograph represents the sheet of sound coming from the transducer. Because the heart is oriented more vertically in the thorax, the sheet of sound needs to be directed more to the tail than the mid lumbar spine, and the transducer needs to be located more cranially and dorsally to be in front of the heart. Short-axis echocardiographic images of the heart have the sheet of sound oriented 90° to the long axis.

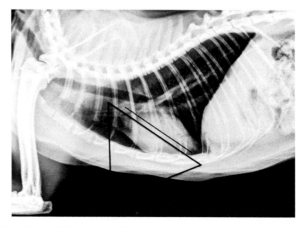

Figure 1.4 Feline lateral thoracic radiograph. This lateral radiograph shows the typical orientation of the cat's heart in the thorax. Note that it is aligned more parallel to the sternum than the dog's heart. The triangle superimposed over this radiograph represents the sheet of sound coming from the transducer. The sheet of sound needs to be directed more towards the thoracolumbar junction than in the dog in order to create the long-axis image. Short-axis echocardiographic images of the heart have the sheet of sound oriented 90° to the long axis.

How To

- Shaving (see Figures 1.5–1.6)
    - If the hair coat is thin enough to see the skin, shaving is not really necessary.
    - Most cats require shaving
    - If shaving is necessary
        - Shave from behind the front leg to about the sixth intercostal space on the right side, from the costochondral junction to the sternum.

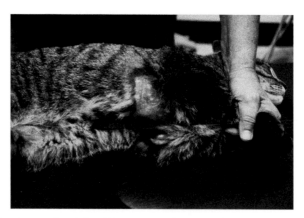

Figure 1.5 Shaving on the right side. On the right side of the thorax in both dogs and cats, shave from behind the front leg to about the sixth intercostal space, from the costochondral junction to the sternum.

○ Shave from behind the front leg at the costochondral junction to just past the last rib on the left side in a triangle shape.

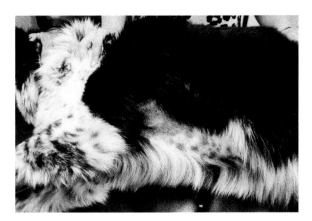

Figure 1.6 Shaving on the left side. On the left side of the thorax in both dogs and cats shave from behind the front leg at the costochondral junction to just past the last rib in a triangular shape. Shaving past the last rib is essential in order to obtain good image quality and long left apical views.

• Use a scan table for the best results (see Figures 1.7–1.8)

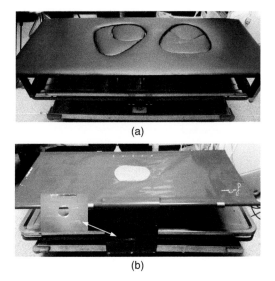

(a)

(b)

Figure 1.7 The Echocardiographic Scan Table. (a–c) A table with cut-outs that allow placement of the transducer from below the thorax enhances image quality because it reduces lung interference. Here, three echo scan tables are seen. (a) A homemade table with various cut-outs for different scanning techniques. (b) A commercially available table with a single cut-out that is used for both left and right parasternal imaging. An overlay (line with arrows) with a smaller hole can be positioned over the larger hole in order to accommodate small dogs and cats. (*Continued*)

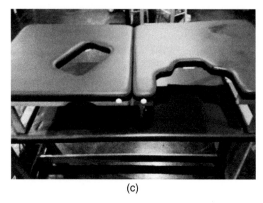

(c)

Figure 1.7 (*Continued*) (c) Another commercially available scan table with cut-outs at each end of the table, one located at the edge of the table for left parasternal imaging. Many other options exist, but all improve image quality and minimize frustration.

- o The heart will drop through the lungs, providing better image quality.
- o Position in right or left lateral recumbency depending upon the imaging plane desired.
- o Place the animal's thorax over the cut-out in the table.

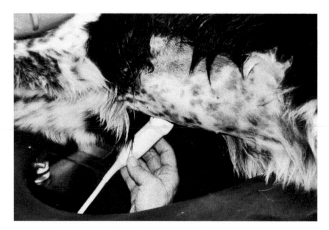

Figure 1.8 The Echocardiographic Scan Table and Animal Placement. Place the animal in right or left lateral recumbency over the table cut-out. Here, the dog is placed in right lateral recumbency on the table with the thorax located over the cut-out. The dog's head is to the left side of this image. The transducer is positioned against the right side of the thorax from below the dog to obtain the right parasternal imaging planes. The heart drops through the lungs, and image quality is generally improved over imaging that is done with the animal placed in left lateral recumbency and obtaining right parasternal images from above. The same principles apply when obtaining left parasternal images: the animal is place left-side down over the cut-out.

Chapter 2 Knobology for the Echocardiogram: Improving Image Quality

Depth

- Adjust depth to fill the entire sector with the heart
- Do not have a lot of useless space below your heart

Two-Dimensional and M-Mode Echocardiography for the Small Animal Practitioner, Second Edition. June A. Boon.
© 2017 John Wiley & Sons, Inc. Published 2017 by John Wiley & Sons, Inc.
Companion Website: www.wiley.com/go/boon/two-dimensional

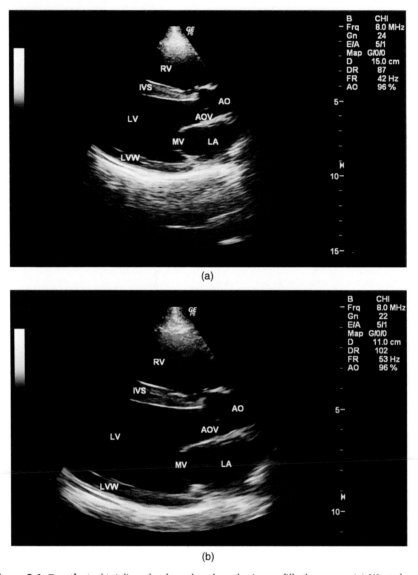

(a)

(b)

Figure 2.1 Depth. (a, b) Adjust depth so that the echo image fills the sector. (a) Wasted space below the image; (b) An appropriate depth setting. For details of abbreviations used in the figures, see the Glossary.

Frequency

- Higher-frequency transducers
  - Have shorter wavelengths
  - Have better resolution
  - Have less depth penetration

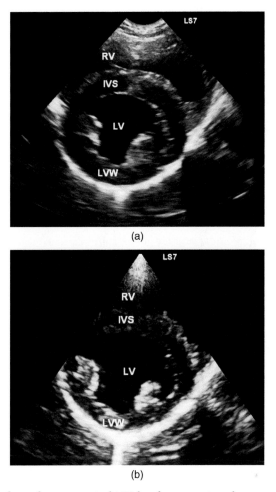

(a)

(b)

Figure 2.2 Transducer frequency. (a, b) Higher-frequency transducers provide better image resolution but less depth penetration, while low-frequency transducers can image deeper structures but have poorer resolution. (a) A high-frequency transducer used in a dog. (b) A lower-frequency transducer used in the same dog. Image quality is poorer in panel (b) than in panel (a).

- Lower-frequency transducers
  - Have longer wavelengths
  - Have poorer resolution
    - Not necessarily noticeable in larger animals where structures are larger
    - Noticeably poorer if used in small hearts
  - More depth penetration
- Use the highest frequency that provides adequate depth
- Some machines have resolution, general and penetration settings

- ○ Resolution is the highest frequency and provides the best quality image but may not go deep enough
- ○ Penetration is the lowest frequency and will go deeper through the thorax but may not give the best image quality in smaller animals
  - Use penetration for large or difficult-to-image animals
- ○ The general setting is somewhere in between resolution and penetration

Gain

- This control increases or decreases brightness of the entire image.
- Adjust gain so that structures are easily seen but not so high that pixels start blurring together.
- Some machines have near and far gain knobs.
  - ○ Near gain controls brightness at the top of the sector – the "near field"
  - ○ Far gain controls brightness at the bottom of the sector – the "far field"
  - ○ These near and far gain controls sometimes replace time gain compensation (TGC) sliders on some machines

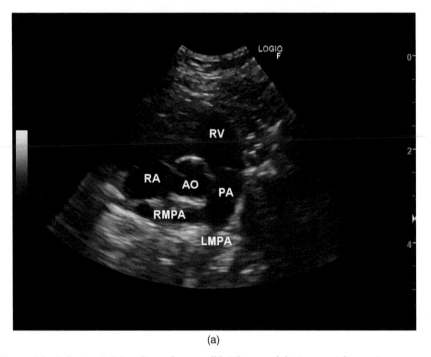

(a)

Figure 2.3 Gain. (a–c) Gain adjusts the overall brightness of the image. Adjust gain to see structures clearly. (a) A low gain setting, where the image is too black and details are difficult to see; (*Continued*)

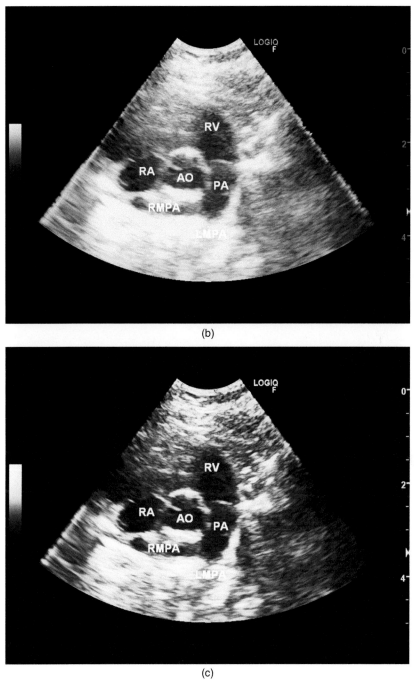

(b)

(c)

Figure 2.3 (*Continued*) (b) A very high gain setting, where the pixels begin to blend together and details are lost. (c) An appropriate gain setting.

Time gain compensation (TGC)

- Sound loses energy as it travels through the thorax
  - This is called attenuation
- Reflections of sound back to the transducer:
  - Are strong in the near field
  - Get weaker with increasing depth
- TGC sliders
  - Each slider controls the gain across the entire sector at a specific depth
  - The goal is to have similar gain settings throughout the entire image from top to bottom
  - Adjust sliders to accomplish this goal
    - Decrease the brightness of strong signals in the near field
      - □ Move sliders left to decrease gain
    - Enhance the brightness of weaker signals in the far field
      - □ Move sliders right to increase gain

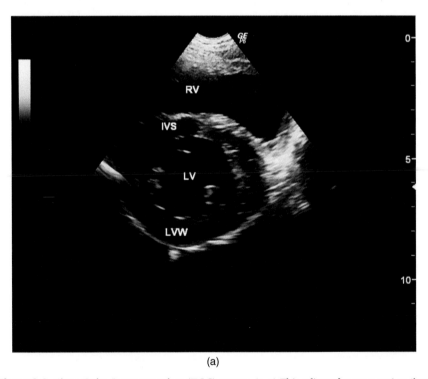

(a)

Figure 2.4 Time Gain Compensation (TGC) curve. (a–c) This adjusts for attenuation (loss of sound energy) as the sound beams travel deeper into the body. Using overall gain would increase gain over the entire image, while TCG sliders control gain at specific depths. (a) Far-field attenuation with low gain. The appropriate TGC sliders should be moved to the right in order to increase brightness at that depth; (*Continued*)

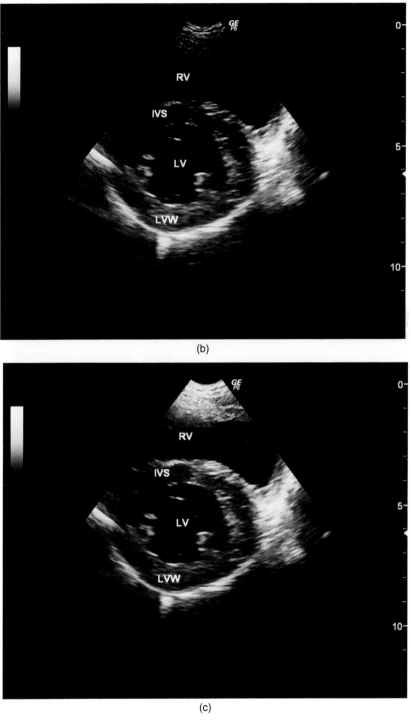

(b)

(c)

Figure 2.4 (*Continued*) (b) Too little gain in the near field; the top few TGC sliders should be moved to the right in order to increase the level of brightness in the near field; (c) The TGC curve adjusted so that gain levels are similar from near to far field.

Grey Map

- Reflected sound is assigned brighter or softer shades of grey, based on the map selected
- Some maps show very soft grays, some show very bright levels of grey
- There is no right or wrong here; select the map based on personal preference but that shows the necessary details
- The default map for your preset should be the one that is used the most and is only adjusted if the image is not pleasing
- Adjusting the grey map may provide better image quality in difficult-to-image animals

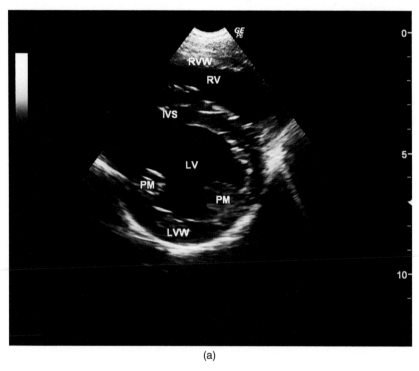

(a)

Figure 2.5 Grey maps. (a, b) Grey maps change the intensity of grays in the image. (a) A gray map with more contrast than in panel (b), which shows softer grays. Adjust based on personal preference without losing image detail.

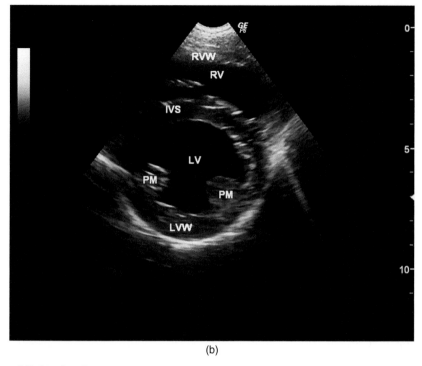

(b)

Figure 2.5 (*Continued*)

Dynamic Range

- This controls how many shades of grey are displayed
- This is sometimes called compression
  - The grey levels are compressed into fewer shades if the dynamic range is low
  - The grey levels are expanded into more shades if the dynamic range is high
- Adjust dynamic range for personal preference without losing image details
- The default dynamic range for your preset should be the one that is used the most, and is only adjusted if the image is not pleasing
- Adjusting the dynamic range may provide better image quality in difficult-to-image animals
- Varying combinations of grey map and dynamic range can result in the same levels of grayness and brightness.
  - It does not matter which is adjusted first

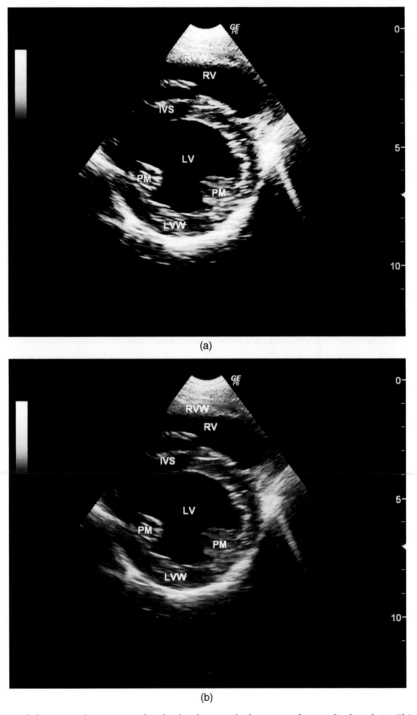

(a)

(b)

Figure 2.6 Dynamic range. (a, b) This knob controls the range of grays displayed. (a) This shows a narrow range of grays; (b) A large range of grays. Select the dynamic range based on personal preference and without loss of image quality.

Rejection

- This button selects the minimum level of sound reflection to be displayed
- Rejection of low-level sound reflections cleans up the background noise
  - Rejection is often used in M-mode images

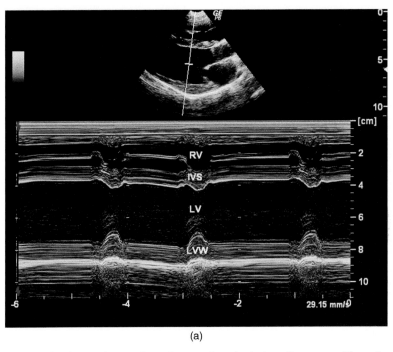

(a)

Figure 2.7 Rejection. (a, b) Low-intensity sound can be "rejected" – removed from the image. (a) An M-mode image without a lot of rejection; (b) The same image with a lot of rejection added; this results in blacker chambers. Here, so much rejection has been added that some details are lost. Rejection is used more often in M-mode imaging than in two-dimensional imaging.

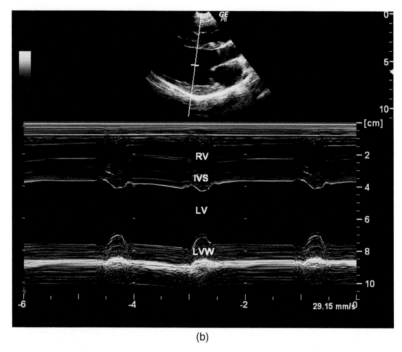

(b)

Figure 2.7 (*Continued*)

Focus

- The focal point improves resolution at the level it is set
- Typically it is positioned in the bottom half to one-third of the sector image but place the focus at any depth as needed to improve image quality at that location
- In cardiac imaging use no more than one focus

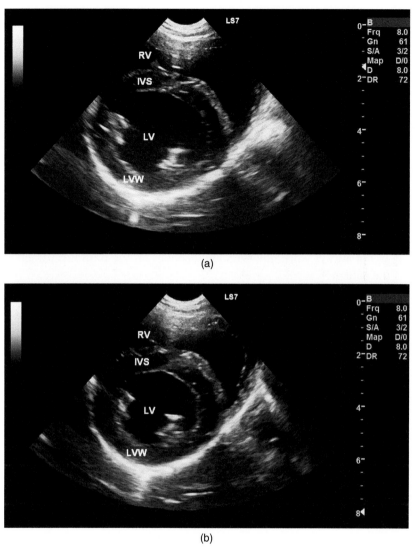

(a)

(b)

Figure 2.8 Focus. (a, b) The focus allows the beam to be narrowed and display better resolution at whatever depth it is placed. Usually, a symbol of some sort along the depth indicators shows where the focus is (triangles). (a) A focus positioned in the near field. (b) The focus is positioned in the bottom half of the image. Overall resolution is better in panel (b), while far-field structures lack good resolution in panel (a). Place the focus in the area of interest or near the bottom one-third of the sector image.

Scan Area

- Also called sector width
- This sets the width of the sector image

- Wider sectors take longer to process and the frame rate decreases
  - Faster heart rates may require smaller sector widths in order to process the image fast enough
  - Small dogs and cats with fast heart rates often require smaller sector widths for good image resolution
  - Sector width is always smaller for echocardiograms than for abdominal scanning

Harmonics

- Harmonic imaging allows the transducer to send sound out at one frequency but receive sound at a higher frequency
- This usually improves image quality and reduces the number of artifacts
- It does not always work however, and depends on the transducer frequency and the patient
  - Turn harmonics on or off and see which setting provides the best quality image

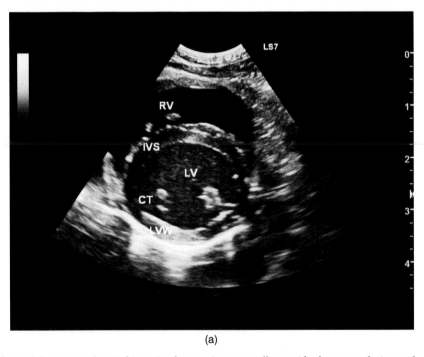

(a)

Figure 2.9 Harmonics. (a, b) Having harmonics on usually provides better resolution and fewer artifacts. It does not always work, however, depending on the transducer frequency and the patient. Turn harmonics on or off and see which setting provides the best image quality. (a) Harmonics on; (b) Harmonics off.

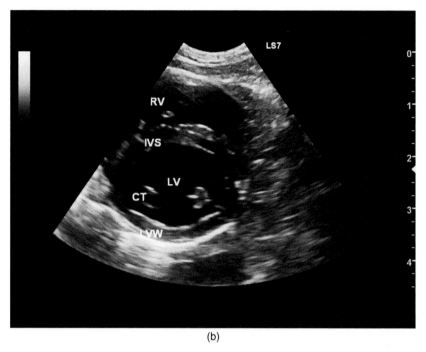

(b)

Figure 2.9 (*Continued*)

Sweep Speed

- This setting is used for M-mode images
- It spreads out the time line
  - Use a sweep speed that allows for easy measuring

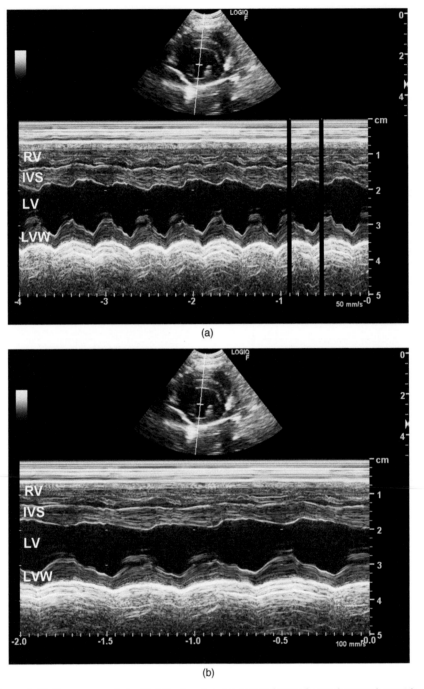

(a)

(b)

Figure 2.10 Sweep speed. (a, b) Adjusting the sweep speed spreads out the time line with faster heart rates and compresses it with slower heart rates. (a) A feline left ventricular M-mode echocardiogram where the cardiac cycles are close together; (b) The same M-mode echocardiogram with a faster sweep speed.

Compounding and Cross Beam

- These controls are not used in cardiac imaging as they decrease the frame rate and prevent the rapid image generation necessary in echocardiography.

Chapter 3 Two-Dimensional Imaging Planes and Subjective Assessment

Two-Dimensional and M-Mode Echocardiography for the Small Animal Practitioner, Second Edition. June A. Boon.
© 2017 John Wiley & Sons, Inc. Published 2017 by John Wiley & Sons, Inc.
Companion Website: www.wiley.com/go/boon/two-dimensional

RIGHT PARASTERNAL IMAGING PLANES: LONG-AXIS VIEWS

Left Ventricular Inflow Outflow (Left Ventricular Outflow)

- Features of the normal left ventricular inflow outflow view in the dog
  - The interventricular septum is straight (see Figure 3.1 and Video 3.1)
    - Upward curvature suggests a dilated left ventricle (see Figure 3.2)
    - Downward curvature suggests one of the following (see Figure 3.3):
      - Left ventricular volume contraction
      - Right ventricular volume and/or pressure overloads

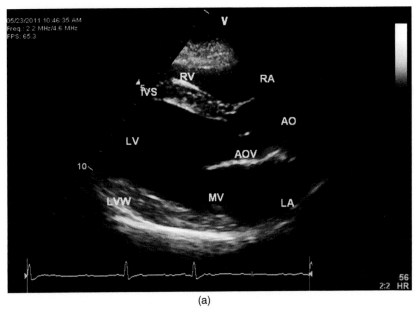

(a)

Video 3.1

Figure 3.1 Normal right parasternal left ventricular inflow outflow view in the dog. (a, b) The ideal long-axis inflow outflow image is horizontal across the sector, has a parallel wall and interventricular septum, has an aorta that shows the aortic valve dash in its middle during diastole, and has a mitral valve that opens well into the left ventricular chamber. (a) In diastole, as seen here, the mitral valve, chamber size, wall thicknesses and left atrial size are assessed. See text for features of the normal inflow outflow view in the dog; (b) In systole, the mitral valve is assessed for prolapse. Here, the mitral valve does not curve backwards into the left atrial chamber. For details of abbreviations used in the figures, see the Glossary.

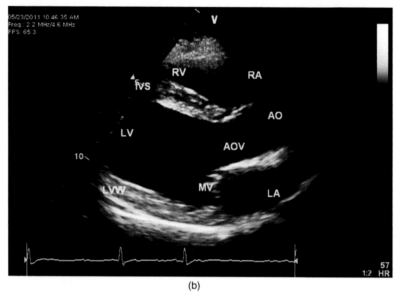

(b)

Figure 3.1 (*Continued*)

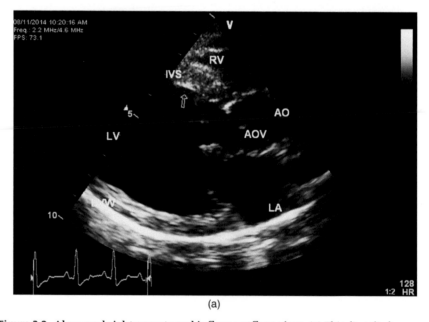

(a)

Figure 3.2 Abnormal right parasternal inflow outflow view. (a) This diastolic frame shows a ventricular septum that curves upward (arrow), consistent with a dilated left ventricular chamber, a left atrium that is larger than the aorta, consistent with left atrial dilation and an anterior mitral valve leaflet that is thickened; (b) This systolic frame shows prolapse (arrow) of the mitral leaflet into the left atrial chamber.

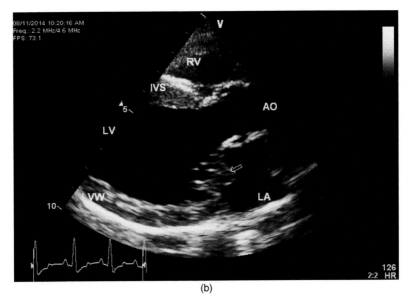

(b)

Figure 3.2 (*Continued*)

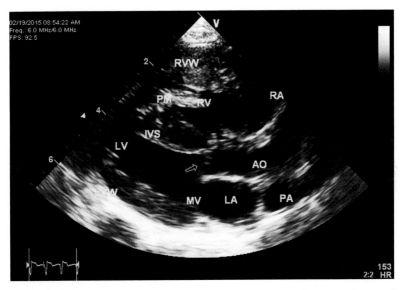

Figure 3.3 Abnormal right parasternal inflow outflow view. This image shows right ventricular hypertrophy with a wall thickness that is much more than left ventricular wall thickness. The pressure overload that is creating this hypertrophy causes the interventricular septum to curve downward. A component of this downwardly curved septum may be secondary to decreased preload in the left ventricular chamber. The result is that the left ventricular walls appear thick because of poor volume in the heart. Only about two wall or septal thicknesses fit in this left ventricular chamber. There is a fibrous band of tissue extending down from the interventricular septum into the left ventricular outflow tract (arrow). This is one finding of subaortic stenosis in the dog which may also be creating the hypertrophic appearance in this heart.

○ The left ventricular wall and interventricular septum are similar in thickness
○ About four wall or septal thicknesses should fill the left ventricular chamber
  ▪ Less than three thicknesses would be consistent with thick left ventricular
    walls (see Figures 3.3 and 3.6)
  ▪ More than five thicknesses would be consistent with left ventricular dila-
    tion and possibly thin walls (see Figure 3.2a)
○ The aorta and left atrium are similar in size
  ▪ An atrium that is much larger than the aorta is dilated (see Figure 3.2)
○ The mitral valve
  ▪ Is thin with the same thickness from the leaflets to their tips during dias-
    tole (see Figures 3.1a and 3.2a)
  ▪ Does not prolapse (bend) back or point into the left atrium during systole
    (see Figure 3.2b)
○ The ventricular septum does not extend down into the left ventricular out-
  flow tract
○ There is no band of tissue in the subvalvular area
  ▪ Septal hypertrophy or fibrous tissue in the outflow tract are seen with
    □ obstruction to left ventricular outflow (see Figure 3.3)
    □ significant volume contraction (see Figure 3.3)
○ The right ventricular chamber is approximately one-third to one-half the
  size of the left ventricular chamber at their largest dimensions (see Fig-
  ures 3.1 and 3.4)

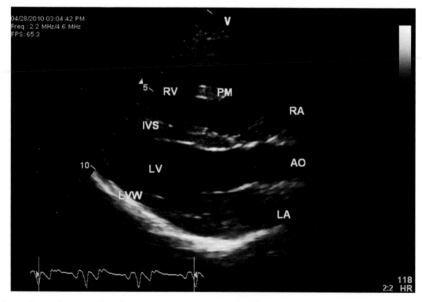

Figure 3.4 Abnormal right parasternal inflow outflow view. This image shows a right
ventricular chamber that is much larger than the left ventricular chamber. The right
ventricular chamber should be about one-third to one-half the size of the left ventricular
chamber.

- ○ The right ventricular wall is approximately one-half the thickness of the left ventricular wall
  - A right ventricular wall as thick or thicker than the left ventricular wall is hypertrophied (see Figure 3.3)
- Features of the normal left ventricular inflow outflow view in the cat (see Figures 3.5–3.6 and Videos 3.5–3.6)

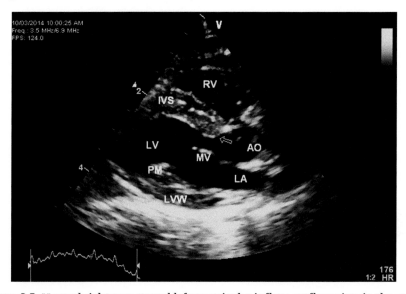

Figure 3.5 Normal right parasternal left ventricular inflow outflow view in the cat.
The ideal long-axis inflow outflow view image is horizontal across the sector, the septum may bow slightly upward at end-diastole, the left atrium may appear larger than the aorta (it is not larger in this image), the interventricular septum may normally extend down in the left ventricular outflow tract to a small degree (arrow), the interventricular septum and wall thicknesses are similar, about three to four wall or septal thicknesses should fit into the left ventricular chamber at end-diastole, the right ventricular chamber should be one-half or less the size of the left ventricular chamber, the right wall thickness should be about one-half the thickness of the normal left ventricular wall.

- ○ The septum may bow *slightly* upward
- ○ The left atrium may appear to be larger than the aorta
  - A left atrium that is much larger than the aorta is consistent with left atrial dilation
- ○ The ventricular septum may normally extend down into the left ventricular outflow tract to a small degree (see Figure 3.5)
- ○ The width of the left ventricular outflow tract should not change as the heart contracts
- ○ Normal mitral valve appearance (see Figures 3.5–3.6a)
  - Thin pliable leaflets with no upward motion during systole
  - Systolic upward (anterior) motion (SAM) during systole is a finding associated with left ventricular outflow obstruction and hypertrophic obstructive cardiomyopathy (see Figure 3.6 and Video 3.6)

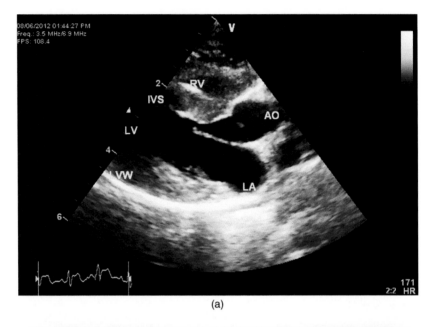

(a)

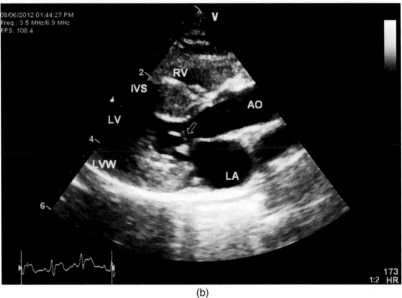

(b)

Video 3.6

Figure 3.6 Abnormal right parasternal left ventricular inflow outflow view in the cat. (a) This long-axis view shows a hypertrophied interventricular septum and wall – only about two of these thicknesses can fit into the left ventricular chamber at end-diastole, the mitral valve is normal with no irregularities during diastole when it is wide open; (b) This long-axis view shows systolic anterior mitral valve motion (SAM) of the mitral valve (arrow). This should not occur, and is a sign of left ventricular outflow tract obstruction.

- The right ventricular wall is about one-half the thickness of the left ventricular wall
  - Make sure the left ventricular wall is normal in thickness, based on measurements
  - If the relationship of right to left wall thickness is normal and the left wall is thick, then so is the right
- The right ventricular chamber is approximately one-third the size of the left ventricular chamber at their largest dimension

Four-Chamber

- Features of the normal four-chamber view in the dog and cat (see Figures 3.7– 3.8 and Videos 3.7–3.8)
  - The interatrial septum is straight
    - An upwardly directed atrial septum suggests left atrial dilation (see Figure 3.9)
    - A downwardly curved atrial septum suggests right atrial dilation (see Figure 3.10)

Video 3.7

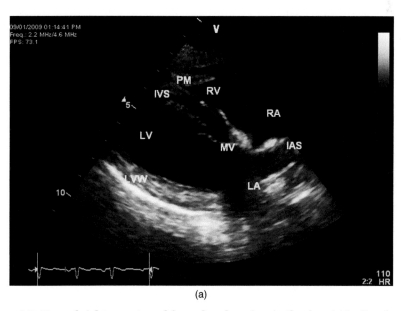

(a)

Figure 3.7 Normal right parasternal four-chamber view in the dog. (a) In diastole, the normal four-chamber view should show an interventricular septum and left ventricular wall that are parallel to each other, an interventricular septum that is straight, an interatrial septum that is straight, and mitral valve leaflets that are thin from the base of the leaflets to their tips; (b) The mitral valve leaflets should not prolapse during systole. The closed leaflets should not break the plane defined by the mitral annulus (hinge points of the leaflets). It is normal to see chordae tendineae extend from the leaflets during systole, and this is the reason why irregularities of the valve are not assessed during systole.

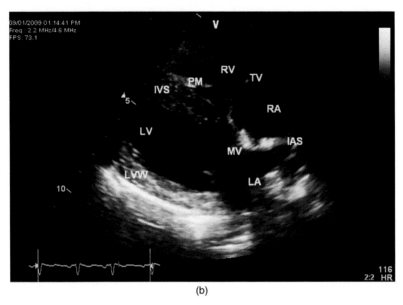

(b)

Figure 3.7 (*Continued*)

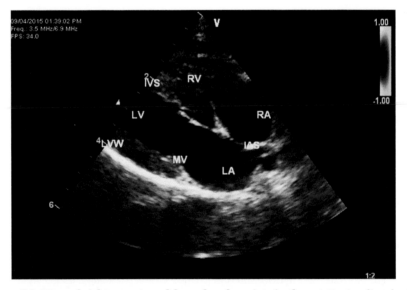

Video 3.8

Figure 3.8 Normal right parasternal four-chamber view in the cat. During diastole, the normal four-chamber view should show an interventricular septum and left ventricular wall that are parallel to each other, an interventricular septum that is straight, an interatrial septum that is straight, and mitral valve leaflets that are thin from the base of the leaflets to their tips.

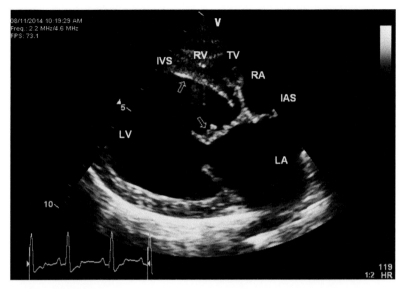

Figure 3.9 Abnormal right parasternal four-chamber view in the dog. This four-chamber view shows a curved interventricular septum (arrow) consistent with left ventricular dilation, a thick and irregular anterior mitral valve leaflet (arrow), and an interatrial septum that is directed upward on the right side of the sector image consistent with left atrial dilation.

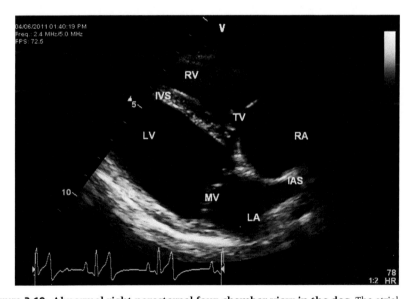

Figure 3.10 Abnormal right parasternal four-chamber view in the dog. The atrial septum is curved downward in the four-chamber view, consistent with right atrial dilation. The right atrium should be similar in size to the left atrium.

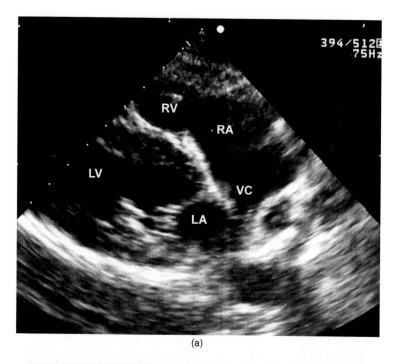

(a)

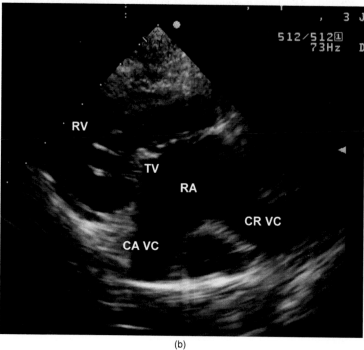

(b)

Figure 3.11 Cranial and caudal vena cava. (a) Lifting the transducer up towards the dog's thorax from the four-chamber view, making the angle between the transducer and the thorax smaller, brings the caudal vena cava into view. This can be mistaken for right atrial dilation. (b) Continuing to lift the transducer up towards the thorax and adding a little rotation will show more of the caudal and the cranial vena cava.

□ If you lift the transducer while obtaining this view the caudal vena cava is seen, and this may make the right atrium appear falsely dilated (see Figure 3.11)
  ○ The ventricular septum is straight (see Figures 3.7–3.8 and Video 3.7)
    ■ The slight upward curve as it moves away from the mitral annulus is normal
    ■ Downward curvature suggests:
      □ Right ventricular dilation
      □ Left ventricular volume contraction
    ■ Upward curvature is consistent with left ventricular dilation (see Figure 3.9)
    ■ The mitral valve leaflets are normal
      □ This is the best right parasternal imaging plane to see lesions without falsely creating them (see Figure 3.9)
  ○ The right ventricular wall thickness is about one-half the thickness of the left ventricular wall thickness (see Figure 3.12)

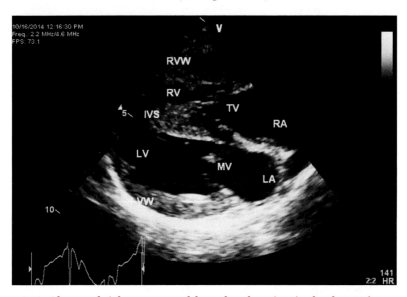

Figure 3.12 Abnormal right parasternal four-chamber view in the dog. Right ventricular wall thickness should be about one-half the thickness of the left ventricular wall in the normal heart. This heart has right ventricular hypertrophy, with a wall thickness that is much thicker than the left ventricular wall. The interventricular septum is also thicker than the left ventricular wall and is part of the right ventricular hypertrophic pattern.

RIGHT PARASTERNAL IMAGING PLANES: SHORT-AXIS (TRANSVERSE) VIEWS

Left Ventricle at the Papillary Muscles

- Features of the normal transverse left ventricle at the papillary muscles in the dog and cat (see Figure 3.13 and Video 3.13)

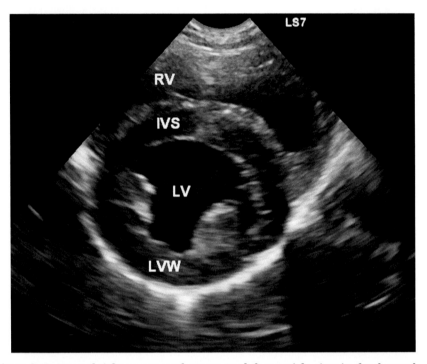

Video 3.13

Figure 3.13 Normal right parasternal transverse left ventricle view in the dog and cat. The normal transverse left ventricular view should have an outer shape that is circular, a left ventricular chamber that is shaped like a mushroom, papillary muscles that are similar in size, and a right ventricular chamber dimension above the septum that is no more than one-third to one-half the size of the left ventricular dimension. A third papillary muscle is a normal finding in both cats and dogs, and is seen on the feline video.

- The outer shape of the left ventricle is symmetrical and circular
- The left ventricular chamber itself is mushroom- shaped
- Papillary muscles are similar in size
  - A third papillary muscle is a normal finding in both dogs and cats (see Video 3.13)
- The ventricular septum is curved up and not flattened (see Figure 3.14–3.15)
  - A flattened septum is seen with right ventricular pressure and volume overloads
- There is uniform contraction of all walls towards the centre of the chamber
- The right ventricular wall thickness is about one-third the thickness of the left ventricular wall thickness (see Figure 3.15)
- Irregularities on the right side of the septum are normal (see Figure 3.16)
  - They represent the trabeculae and papillary muscles of the right ventricle

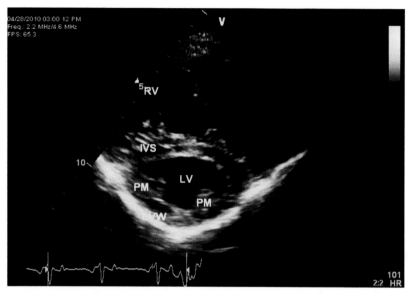

Figure 3.14 Abnormal right parasternal transverse left ventricle view. A flattened ventricular septum occurs when the right ventricular chamber is either dilated or hypertrophied secondary to volume or pressure overload. Here, the septum is flattened because of right ventricular volume overload.

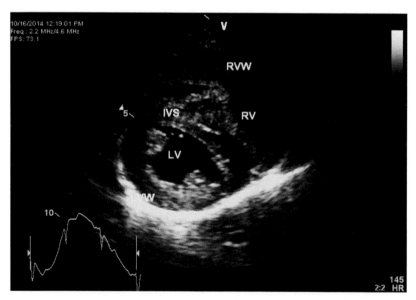

Figure 3.15 Abnormal right parasternal transverse left ventricle view. The right ventricular wall should be no more than one-half the thickness of the left ventricular wall. Right ventricular hypertrophy occurs secondary to pressure overload because of pulmonary hypertension or pulmonic stenosis. Here, the left ventricular wall and septum also appear thick because of poor preload in the left ventricular chamber.

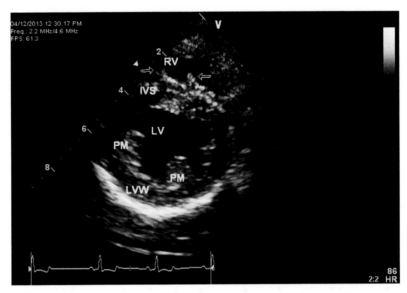

Figure 3.16 Normal right parasternal transverse left ventricle view. Irregularities (arrows) on the right ventricular side of the interventricular septum are a normal finding. They represent the trabeculae found in the right side of the heart.

Left Ventricle at the Chordae Tendineae

- Features of the normal transverse left ventricle at the chordae tendineae in the dog and cat (see Figure 3.17 and Video 3.17)

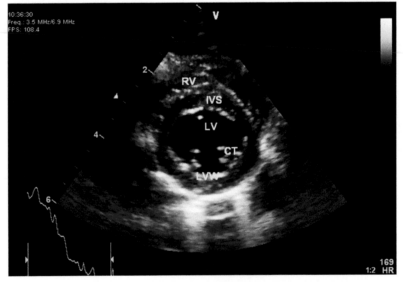

Video 3.17

Figure 3.17 Normal right parasternal transverse chordae tendineae view. Bright white lines seen where the papillary muscles used to be represent the chordae tendineae on the transverse view in a cat. This is the level at which left ventricular measurements are made.

- o The outer shape of the left ventricle is a symmetrical circle
- o Bright lines replace the muscular bundles of the papillary muscles
- o This is the view used to make left ventricular measurements

Left Ventricle at the Mitral valve

- Features of the normal transverse left ventricle at the mitral valve in the dog and cat (see Figure 3.18 and Video 3.18)
  - o No reliable subjective assessment on this view
  - o Mitral valve leaflets can falsely appear irregular on this view
  - o The leaflets should move well away from each other and are often called a "fish mouth"

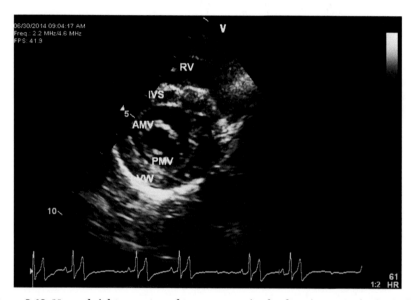

Figure 3.18 Normal right parasternal transverse mitral valve view. Mitral valve leaflets move away from each other during diastole, with the anterior leaflet moving up towards the interventricular septum and the posterior leaflet moving down towards the left ventricular wall. The leaflets move towards each other during systole. This view is often called the "fish mouth" view.

Video 3.18

Heart Base: At the Left Atrium

- Features of the normal transverse heart base at the left atrium in the dog and cat (see Figure 3.19 and Video 3.19)
  - o The aorta and left atrium are similar in size
  - o The left atrium in cats often looks slightly larger than the aorta

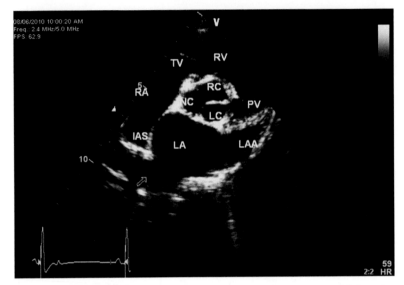

Video 3.19

Figure 3.19 Normal right parasternal transverse heart base: aorta and left atrium view. The aorta is a circular or clover-shaped structure in the middle of the sector image. The junctions of the three aortic valve cusps which are seen are often called the "Mercedes" sign. The left atrium is below the aorta, and to the right side is the left atrial appendage. The aorta and left atrial chamber should appear to be similar in size during the cardiac cycles. Frame-by-frame analysis shows an atrial chamber that is about 1.5-fold larger than the aorta at end-systole, when the atrial size is at its maximum in both cats and dogs. The right side of the heart is seen at the top of the sector image, but subjective assessment of the tricuspid valve and any pulmonary valve that is seen is limited. A pulmonary vein is often seen entering the left atrial chamber (arrow).

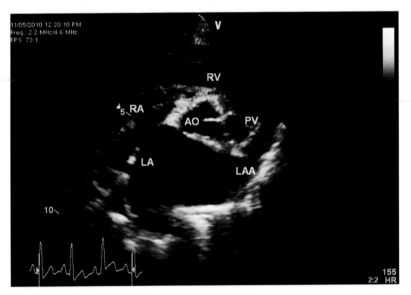

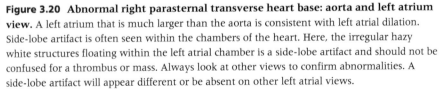
Video 3.20

Figure 3.20 Abnormal right parasternal transverse heart base: aorta and left atrium view. A left atrium that is much larger than the aorta is consistent with left atrial dilation. Side-lobe artifact is often seen within the chambers of the heart. Here, the irregular hazy white structures floating within the left atrial chamber is a side-lobe artifact and should not be confused for a thrombus or mass. Always look at other views to confirm abnormalities. A side-lobe artifact will appear different or be absent on other left atrial views.

- ■ All three cusps of the aortic valve should be visible (the "Mercedes" sign) and the aorta should be a closed circle when making this comparison
- ■ An atrium that is much larger than the aorta is dilated (see Figure 3.20 and Video 3.20)
  - ○ The left atrial wall makes a smooth transition into the left auricle
  - ○ The left atrial appendage is a clear fluid-filled space with no evidence of a thrombus (see Figure 3.21)

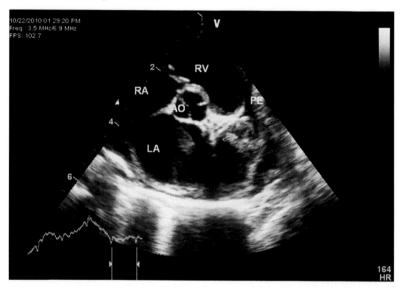

Figure 3.21 Abnormal right parasternal transverse heart base: aorta and left atrium view. A soft-tissue structure within the left atrial appendage (arrow) is consistent with a thrombus in cats. This image also shows some pericardial effusion and a large left atrium.

- ■ A soft-tissue structure in the auricle usually represents a thrombus in the cat – be sure to scan left cranial views of the auricle to confirm this diagnosis
- ■ Side-lobe artifact which usually has a vague indistinct shape should not be confused for thrombus (see Figure 3.20 and Video 3.20)

Heart Base: At the Pulmonary Artery

- • Features of the normal transverse heart base at the pulmonary artery in the dog and cat (see Figure 3.22 and Video 3.22)
  - ○ The aorta and pulmonary artery are similar in diameter
  - ○ The pulmonary artery remains the same width from the level of the valve down to the bifurcation into the right and left branches
    - ■ A pulmonary artery that is wider than the aorta is dilated (see Figure 3.23)
  - ○ The left main pulmonary artery is just barely seen
  - ○ The pulmonary valve cusps move well towards the walls of the pulmonary artery

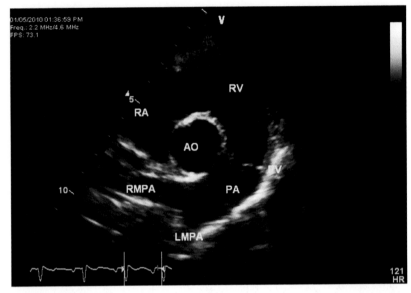

Figure 3.22 Normal right parasternal transverse heart base: aorta and pulmonary artery view. This view is used to assess pulmonary artery size and pulmonary valve motion. The main pulmonary artery should be similar in diameter to the aorta and remain the same size from the pulmonary valve to the bifurcation. The pulmonary valve cusps should move completely to the walls of the artery during systole.

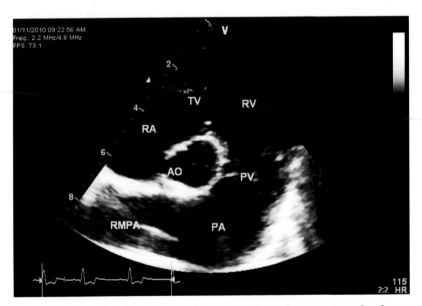

Figure 3.23 Abnormal right parasternal transverse heart base: aorta and pulmonary artery view. This pulmonary artery is much wider than the diameter of the aorta. This finding is consistent with pulmonary hypertension or a shunt.

LEFT PARASTERNAL IMAGING PLANES: CRANIAL LONG-AXIS VIEWS

Left Ventricular Outflow

- Features of the normal left cranial long-axis outflow view in the dog and cat (see Figure 3.24 and Video 3.24)
  - The left ventricular outflow tract should be clear of obstruction (no tissue or muscle)
  - The aortic valve cusps are free of lesions
  - The aorta remains the same diameter all along its length

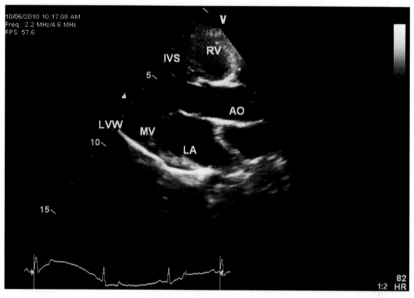

Figure 3.24 Normal left cranial long-axis view of the left ventricular outflow tract. The left ventricular outflow tract should be clear of obstruction, the aortic valves cusps free of lesions, and the aorta should remain the same diameter all along its length. The aortic valve cusps are wide open. The ideal aorta should be somewhat horizontal along the sector image as this is the "echo window" to getting the best right auricle.

Video 3.24

Right Atrium and Auricle

- Features of the normal right atrium and auricle view in the dog and cat (see Figure 3.25 and Video 3.25)
  - The auricle should be clear of soft-tissue densities
  - A soft-tissue structure within or attached to the outside of the atrial appendage is typically consistent with a mass in a dog and thrombus in the cat (see Figure 3.26)

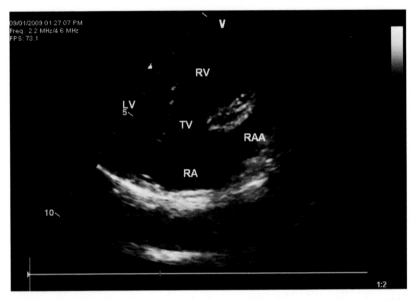

Video 3.25

Figure 3.25 Normal left cranial long-axis view of the right auricle. The normal left cranial long-axis view of the right atrial appendage should show an echo-free space. The bright area above the right auricle and extending to the tricuspid valve is the normal appearance of the myocardium and fat between the right atrial appendage and the right ventricular chamber. This junction can be much larger than this and still be normal.

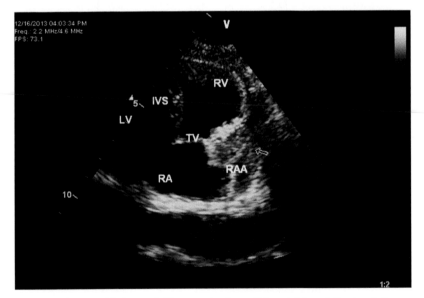

Figure 3.26 Abnormal left cranial long-axis view of the right auricle. A soft-tissue structure (arrow) is seen within the right atrial appendage of this dog. This is consistent with neoplasia, most likely hemangiosarcoma, although other forms of neoplasia and thrombus cannot be completely ruled out.

Pulmonary Artery

- Features of the normal pulmonary artery view in the dog and cat (see Figure 3.27 and Video 3.27)
  - The pulmonic valve should look thin and move well towards the walls of the pulmonary artery
  - There should be no dilation or widening of the artery beyond the valve
  - This is primarily a Doppler view

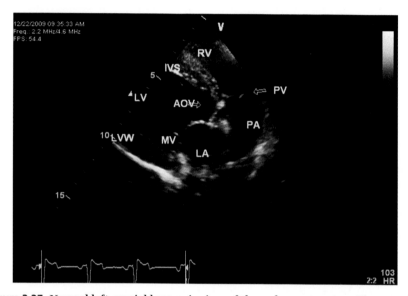

Figure 3.27 Normal left cranial long-axis view of the pulmonary artery. The normal left cranial long-axis of the pulmonary artery (right ventricular outflow tract) shows portions of the left side of the heart and the pulmonary artery to the right side of the sector image. The pulmonary artery bifurcation is typically not seen on this view. The artery should be similar in diameter to the aorta, and the pulmonary valve (arrow) should move well towards the walls of the artery. This is primarily a Doppler view.

Video 3.27

LEFT PARASTERNAL IMAGING PLANES: CRANIAL TRANSVERSE VIEWS

Pulmonary Artery and Tricuspid Valve

- Features of the normal cranial transverse view in the dog and cat (see Figure 3.28 and Video 3.28)
  - The tricuspid valve should move well and look thin in this imaging plane
  - The pulmonary valve should be thin and move well towards the walls of the pulmonary artery

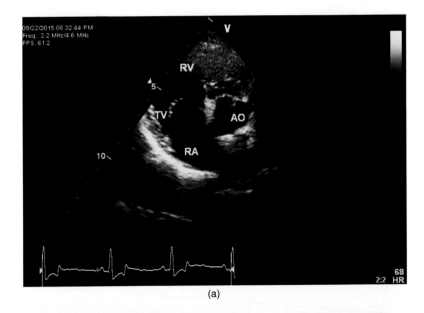

(a)

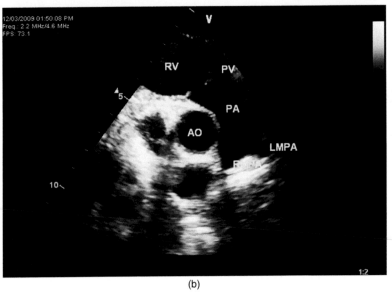

(b)

Video 3.28

Figure 3.28 Normal left cranial transverse view of the heart base. (a,b) The transverse view at the left cranial heart base shows an aorta in the middle of the sector image, below the right ventricular chamber. The right atrium is to the left side of the aorta and the tricuspid valve leaflets open up towards the right ventricular chamber (Figure 3.28a and Video 3.28a). The pulmonary valve is to the right side of the aorta and the main pulmonary artery extends down to the bottom of the sector image (Figure 3.28b and Video 3.28b). The pulmonary artery bifurcation is seen on this imaging plane. The pulmonary artery should be similar in diameter to the aorta and remain the same diameter up to the bifurcation. This is primarily a Doppler view used for pulmonary artery systolic forward and diastolic regurgitant flow and tricuspid regurgitant flow. Often, it is difficult to obtain both the tricuspid valve with good motion and the pulmonary artery in one plane (Figure 3.28c), so each is recorded and viewed separately, as is seen here and in Video 3.28 where the transducer is fanned from the pulmonary artery into the right atrium.

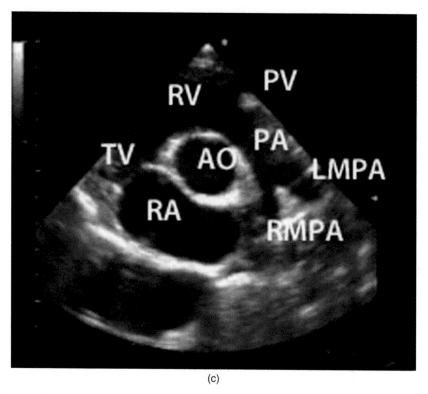
(c)

Figure 3.28 (*Continued*)

- ○ The diameter of the artery should remain the same up to the bifurcation
- ○ This is primarily a Doppler view for pulmonary artery systolic flow, pulmonary insufficiency and tricuspid regurgitation

Heart Base of the Left Auricle

- Features of the normal left auricle view in the cat (see Figure 3.29 and Video 3.29)
  - ○ The auricle should be free from soft-tissue structures
  - ○ A soft-tissue structure or swirling echoes in the auricle of a cat are consistent with thrombus or stasis of blood (see Figure 3.30)

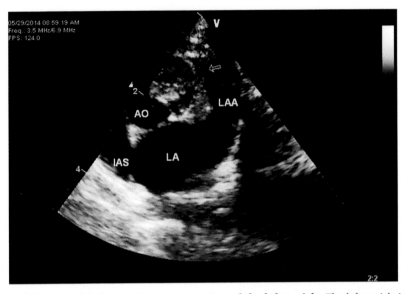

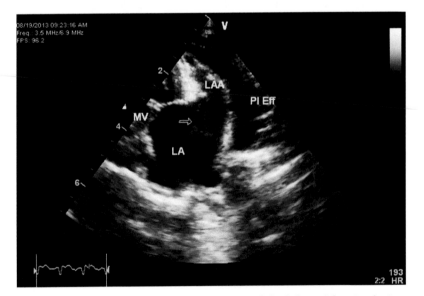

Figure 3.29 Normal left cranial transverse view of the left auricle. The left auricle is seen as you fan caudal from the pulmonary artery on the left cranial transverse view. It is used in cats to see more of the left auricle than is typically seen on right parasternal views of the left auricle. In this video loop, the pulmonary artery is first seen; then, as the transducer is fanned caudally, the left auricle comes into view (arrow). The auricle should be an echo-free space without thrombus. This view often shows "smoke" more readily than right parasternal images of the left atrium. This is primarily a feline view.

Video 3.29

Figure 3.30 Abnormal left cranial transverse view of the left auricle. "Smoke," spontaneous echo contrast, is seen swirling around in this left atrial chamber (arrow). Often, "smoke" is appreciated better on the left cranial view of the left atrium and auricle. There is pleural effusion.

LEFT PARASTERNAL IMAGING PLANES: APICAL VIEWS

Apical Four-Chamber

- Features of the normal left apical four-chamber view in the dog and cat (see Figure 3.31 and Video 3.31)
    - A good apical view has a left ventricular chamber that is about twice as long as it is wide
    - The right atrium is usually smaller or equal in size to the left atrium, but should not be larger than the left atrium
    - Thin smooth mitral valve leaflets with no prolapse
    - This view often shows prolapse and irregularities best
    - This is primarily a Doppler view

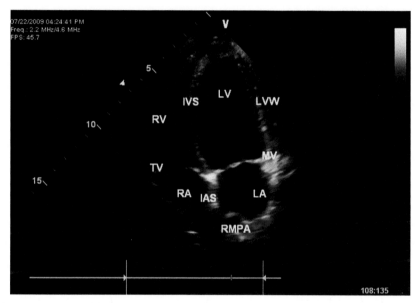

Video 3.31

Figure 3.31 Normal left apical four-chamber view. The apex of the heart is at the top of this left apical image. The left ventricle is to the right, while the right ventricle is to the left side of this sector image. The respective atrial chambers are at the bottom of the sector image. The mitral valve is seen opening up towards the left ventricle on the right side of the sector, while the tricuspid valve is seen between the right atrium and right ventricle on the left side of the sector image. Atrial sizes may be similar in this view, but often the left atrium appears larger because of the way the image is generated. If a very apical view is not obtained the interventricular septum has a slight curve to the right. A good apical view has a left ventricular chamber whose length is about twice as long as its width. The mitral and tricuspid valves should be thin with no prolapse. Although the valves can be assessed on this imaging plane this is primarily a Doppler view for transmitral valve flow and regurgitant jets of both atrioventricular valves.

Apical Five-Chamber

- Features of the normal left apical five-chamber view in the dog and cat (see Figure 3.32 and Video 3.32)

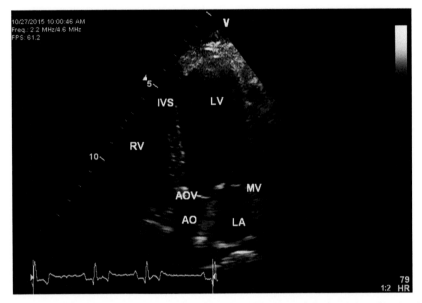

Figure 3.32 Normal left apical five-chamber view. The apex of the heart is at the top of this left apical image. The left ventricle is to the right, while the right ventricle is to the left side of this sector image. The respective atrial chambers are at the bottom of the sector image. The mitral valve will open up towards the left ventricle on the right side of the sector, while the tricuspid valve is not as prominent or visible on this imaging plane. This is because when a good aorta is obtained it is seen at the expense of the right atrium. If a very apical view is not obtained the interventricular septum has a slight curve to the right. A good apical view has a left ventricular chamber whose length is about twice as long as its width. The mitral valve should be thin with no prolapse, and the left ventricular outflow tract should be clear of any soft-tissue structures or hypertrophy of the interventricular septum. Although the valves and subvalvular area of the aorta can be assessed on this imaging plane, this is primarily a Doppler view for transmitral valve flow and regurgitant jets of both atrioventricular valves.

- Although this is referred to as a five-chamber view, the right atrium is not always seen well
- A good apical view has a left ventricular chamber that is about twice as long as it is wide
- Thin smooth mitral valve leaflets with no prolapse
- The left atrium is always larger than the aorta in this plane
- This is primarily a Doppler view

Chapter 4 Imaging Planes: Technique in the Dog and Cat

Two-Dimensional and M-Mode Echocardiography for the Small Animal Practitioner, Second Edition. June A. Boon.
© 2017 John Wiley & Sons, Inc. Published 2017 by John Wiley & Sons, Inc.
Companion Website: www.wiley.com/go/boon/two-dimensional

RIGHT PARASTERNAL IMAGING PLANES: LONG-AXIS VIEWS

Inflow Outflow (Left Ventricular Outflow)

Video 4.1

- Technique in the dog
  - Place the dog in right lateral recumbency over a cut-out in an examination table, with the area of the heart over the cut-out
  - Hold the transducer in the following manner (see Figure 4.1 and Video 4.1):
    - Crystals point towards the lumbar spine
    - Reference mark directed towards the top of the shoulder blades – at the heart base
    - Angle of about 45° between the chest wall and the transducer
  - Without changing how you are holding the transducer, place the transducer in the dog's axilla near the costochondral junction where there is only white haze – no heart
  - Slide in that intercostal space toward the sternum
  - If you do not see a good-quality image of the heart, move caudal one intercostal space and slide up to the costochondral junction
  - Continue this search intercostal space by intercostal space until a good-quality, long-axis image of the heart appears
    - Do not stop the search until you have found the best quality spot
    - It may not be the perfect long-axis plane but it should be the best quality you can find
  - By starting cranially you can find the long axis in its most horizontal position – not an angled view; this will allow you to measure the cardiac chambers and wall thicknesses accurately
  - To perfect the image:
    - If the heart is tipped (apex up) on the sector (see Figure 4.2 and Video 4.1):
      - This means the transducer is located too close to the apex of the heart
      - Slide cranial one intercostal space, dorsal a centimeter or two (more in a large dog, less in a small dog) and point caudal towards the lumbar spine or tail
    - If the left ventricle is not long and the wall and septum are not parallel to each other (see Figure 4.3 and Video 4.1):
      - Twist clockwise or counterclockwise to lengthen the left ventricular chamber – one way or the other will work
    - If the heart base is not seen well and the mitral valve does not open well into the left ventricular chamber (Video 4.1):
      - Lift the transducer up and down without changing where it is pointing (typically the lumbar spine)

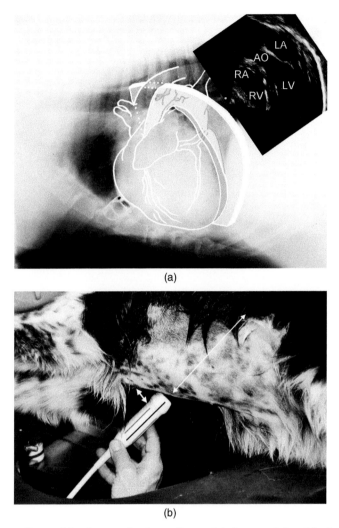

(a)

(b)

Figure 4.1 Radiographic plane and echocardiographic image of the right long-axis inflow outflow view. (a) The transducer is under the dog on the right side of the thorax with the dog placed in right lateral recumbency over a hole in the scan table. The transducer is positioned in front of the heart, pointing caudal as shown here. The sheet of sound is oriented along the length of the heart through the aorta. The corresponding echocardiographic imaging plane is shown to the top right in the same orientation as the sound plane through the thorax. **Transducer position for the right parasternal long-axis inflow outflow view.** (b) The transducer is placed on the right side of the thorax, in front of the heart. The reference mark is opposite the black line and directed towards the heart base at about the top of the shoulder blades. The crystals (the surface of the transducer) are pointed at the lumbar spine (long double-headed arrow) and there should be an angle of about 45° between the transducer and the chest wall (short white double-arrow line). For details of abbreviations used in the figures, see the Glossary.

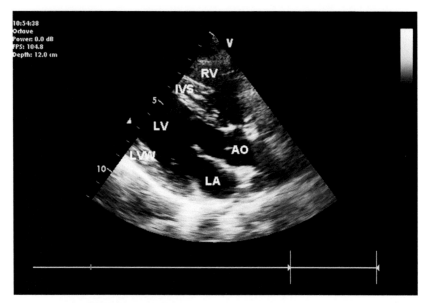

Figure 4.2 An angled inflow outflow view. This is an angled (apex up, base down) long-axis inflow outflow view. This image is appropriate for subjective assessment and color flow Doppler, but should be oriented more horizontally across the sector image in order to obtain accurate measurements of size. See the text and Video 4.1 for instructions on how to achieve a more horizontally oriented imaging plane.

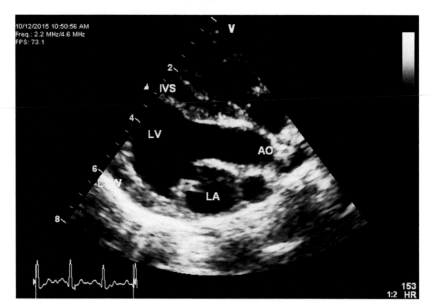

Figure 4.3 A short long-axis inflow outflow view. The wall and septum are not parallel to each other in this inflow outflow view. This is not the longest and widest left ventricular chamber. See the text and Video 4.1 for instructions on how to get a longer and wider left ventricular chamber.

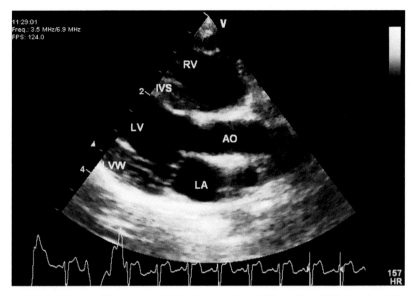

Figure 4.4 Inflow outflow view with left ventricle off the edge of the sector. When either the apex of the heart or the base of the heart are off the sector to the left or right, respectively, the crystals need to be pointed more towards the part of the heart that is not on the sector. In this image the ventricular chambers are only about half-way on the sector, so the transducer needs to be pointed more towards the apex (xyphoid) in order to bring that part of the heart into the sector image.

- If the heart base is off the sector to the right:
  - Point the crystals more cranial towards the heart base
- If most of the left ventricular chamber is off the sector to the left (see Figure 4.4)
  - Point the crystals more towards the xyphoid (the apex of the heart)
- If these movements do not result in a good long-axis outflow image, then you must slide slightly dorsal or ventral in the intercostal space because it implies you are not under the heart properly
  - Follow the steps above to perfect the image again after repositioning in the space
- Modifications in Technique for the Cat
  - Place the cat in right lateral recumbency over a cut-out in an examination table – the sternum only needs to be slightly over the hole as feline hearts sit close to the sternum.
  - Keep the animal's back straight
  - Hold the transducer at about a 45° angle with respect to the chest wall, reference mark to the top of the humerus, and direct the crystals slightly more towards the thoracic spine (see Figures 1.4 and 4.5 and Video 4.2).
    - Start with the transducer way up under the right leg of the cat, right next to the sternum – you should not see the heart yet

Video 4.2

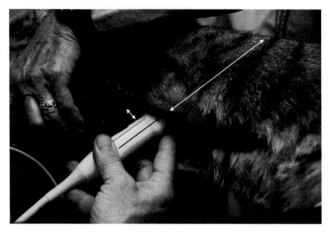

Figure 4.5 Transducer position for the right parasternal long-axis inflow outflow view in the cat. The transducer is placed on the right side of the thorax, in front of the heart. The reference mark is opposite the black line and directed towards the heart base. The crystals (the surface of the transducer) are pointed at the thoracolumbar junction (long double-headed arrow) and there should be an angle of about 45° between the transducer and the chest wall (short white double-arrow line). The crystals are not directed as caudally as in the dog.

- Slide caudally along the sternum with the transducer until you see something beating
- Continue to slide caudal until the beating structure – even if it is hazy – is centered on the monitor
- Stop there and slide (without changing the transducer orientation) to the sternum or the spine in that intercostal space
- One way or the other will show an almost perfect long-axis image of the heart
- Adjust the imaging plane as directed above in the dog – movements are very slight

Four-Chamber

Video 4.3

- Technique in the dog and cat (see Figure 4.6 and Video 4.3)
  - Start with a good left ventricular inflow outflow view
    - Twist the transducer so the reference mark moves away from you toward the spine (see Video 4.3)
    - Do not lift or drop the transducer while twisting until the aorta has disappeared
    - The secret is to never lose mitral valve motion

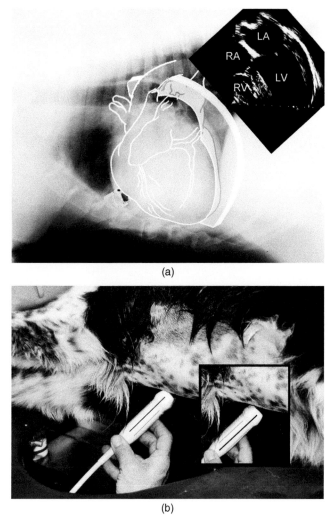

(a)

(b)

Figure 4.6 Radiographic plane and echocardiographic image of the right long-axis four-chamber view. (a) The transducer is under the dog on the right side of the thorax, with the dog placed in right lateral recumbency over a hole in the scan table. The transducer is positioned in front of the heart pointing back at it, as shown here. The sheet of sound is oriented along the length of the heart behind the aorta. This is a subtle rotation of the transducer away from the inflow outflow view. The corresponding echocardiographic imaging plane is shown to the top right in the same orientation as the sound plane through the thorax. **Transducer position for the right parasternal long-axis four-chamber view.** (b) The transducer is placed on the right side of the thorax, in front of the heart. The reference mark is opposite the black line and directed towards the heart base at about the top of the shoulder blades, but rotated towards the spine away from where it was for the inflow outflow view. The smaller inset shows the transducer for the inflow outflow view (note how the reference mark has moved). The crystals (the surface of the transducer) remain pointed at the lumbar spine, and there should be an angle of about 45° between the transducer and the chest wall.

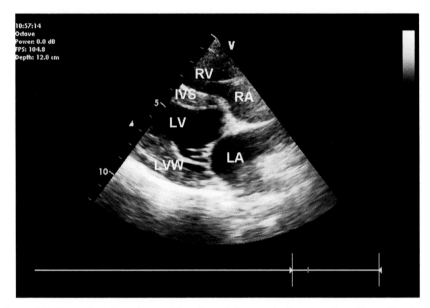

10:57:14
Octave
Power: 0.0 dB
FPS: 104.8
Depth: 12.0 cm

V

RV

IVS   RA

5

LV

LVW   LA

10

Figure 4.7 Four-chamber view with a short left ventricular chamber. The wall and septum are not parallel to each other in this four-chamber view. This is caused by changing the angle between the transducer and the thorax. Do not lift or drop the transducer while twisting away from the inflow outflow view until the aorta has disappeared. The secret is to never lose mitral valve motion.

> □ If mitral valve motion becomes reduced, stop and lift or drop the trans-
> ducer (without changing where you are pointing the crystals) until it
> moves well again, then continue rotating
> - To perfect the image:
>   - Short left ventricular and poor interatrial septum (see Figure 4.7)
>   □ Do not lift or drop the transducer while twisting until the aorta has
>   disappeared
>   □ The secret is to never lose mitral valve motion
>   - If the first imaging plane obtained is the four-chamber view and it does
>   not become an inflow outflow view when rotating the transducer away
>   from the four-chamber view
>   □ The four chamber view was probably obtained with the transducer ori-
>   ented perpendicular to the chest wall
>   □ Start over and obtain a long axis view with the transducer oriented 45°
>   to the chest wall.
>   - The vena cava comes into view (see Figure 3.11)
>   □ The angle between the transducer and the thorax has become smaller
>   □ Drop the transducer down slightly until the atrial septum is seen and
>   the vena cava disappears
>   - The heart is off the sector to the right or left (see Figure 4.4)

     □ Point the crystals toward the thoracic spine in order to bring the heart
base into the sector and towards the xyphoid to see more of the ventricular chambers.

SHORT-AXIS (TRANSVERSE) VIEWS

Technique in the Dog and Cat

- Start with a good left ventricular inflow outflow or four-chamber view
  - Pay attention to the long axis of the heart and how it is aligned within the
thorax (look at your transducer to see how it is oriented along the long axis
when you have it)
  - This line is how you will fan and point the crystals as you move from base
to apex to obtain these transverse views (see Figure 4.8)

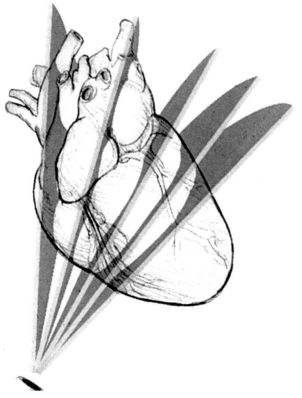

Figure 4.8 Transverse imaging planes. The sound beam is oriented 90° away from the
long-axis planes and the transducer is fanned from base to apex through all the transverse
imaging planes of the heart. Transducer location on the thorax remains the same.

■ Twist the transducer so the reference mark moves away from the spine towards the animal's elbows (see Figure 4.9 and Video 4.4)

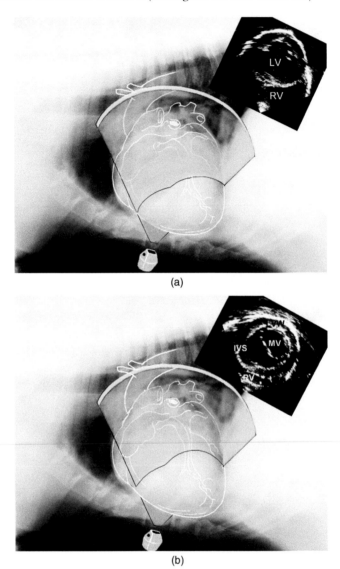

(a)

(b)

Figure 4.9 Radiographic planes and echocardiographic images of the right transverse views. (a–d) The transducer has been rotated 90° from the long-axis plane and is directed through the short-axis planes of the heart. (a) The sheet of sound is directed towards the apex of the heart through the papillary muscles. The corresponding echocardiographic imaging plane is shown to the top right in the same orientation as the sound plane through the thorax. (b) The sheet of sound is directed slightly away from the apex of the heart through the mitral valve. The corresponding echocardiographic imaging plane is shown to the top right in the same orientation as the sound plane through the thorax.

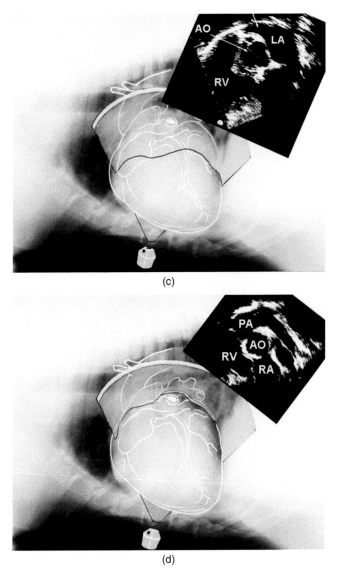

(c)

(d)

Figure 4.9 (*Continued*) (c) The sheet of sound is directed further towards the heart base through the aorta and left atrium. The corresponding echocardiographic imaging plane is shown to the top right in the same orientation as the sound plane through the thorax. (d) The sheet of sound is directed even further towards the heart base through the aorta and pulmonary artery. The corresponding echocardiographic imaging plane is shown to the top right in the same orientation as the sound plane through the thorax.

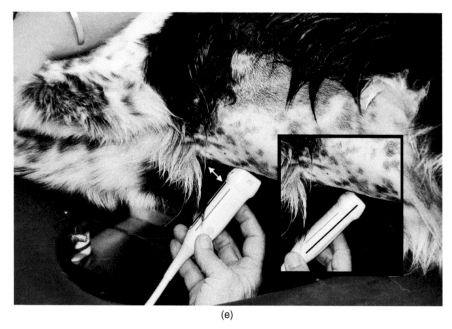

(e)

Figure 4.9 (*Continued*) **Transducer position for the right parasternal short-axis views of the heart.** (e) The transducer is placed on the right side of the thorax, in front of the heart. The reference mark is directed towards the elbows. The smaller inset shows the transducer for the inflow outflow view (note how the reference mark has moved). There should still be an angle of about 45° between the transducer and the chest wall.

- ☐ Do not drop the transducer – keep that at a 45–60° angle between the transducer and the thorax
  - ■ Twist until a round left ventricular chamber or aorta is seen – about 90° from the long-axis plane (see Figure 4.9(e))
- ○ Fan the transducer without rotating so that the crystals point from the base of the heart to the apex along the long axis of the heart (see Figures 4.9 (a–d) and Figure 4.8)
- ○ To perfect the image:
  - ■ The left ventricle is egg-shaped (see Figure 4.10 and Video 4.3)
    - ☐ Rotate the transducer clockwise or counterclockwise until the left ventricle is circular
  - ■ The short-axis view is not completely in the sector, part of it is off the sector to the right or left (see Figure 4.11)
    - ☐ Fan the transducer in the direction of the reference mark or in the direction opposite the reference mark, without changing anything else in order to swing the image right or left across the screen
  - ■ The atrial septum on the LA/AO view is straight out at 9:00 o'clock (see Figure 4.12)
    - ☐ This means the transducer is rotated beyond the transverse plane

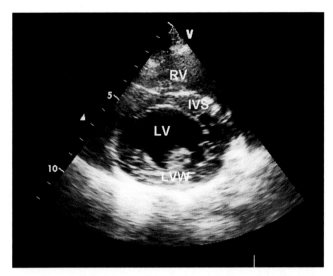

Figure 4.10 An asymmetrical transverse left ventricular chamber. This left ventricle is egg-shaped as opposed to round with symmetrical and equally shaped papillary muscles. See Video 4.3 and the text for directions to fix this.

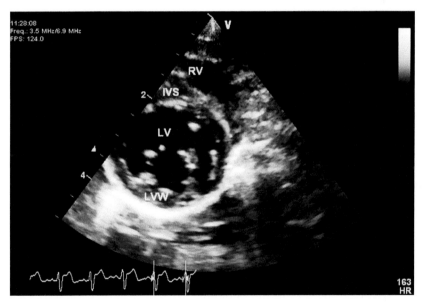

Figure 4.11 Short axis not completely within sector. When any short-axis view is not completely within the sector, partly off the sector to the right or left, the transducer angle needs to change. Fan the transducer in the direction of the reference mark or away from it, changing the angle of the transducer with respect to the thorax. This will swing the heart right or left across the sector image. Do not rotate the transducer.

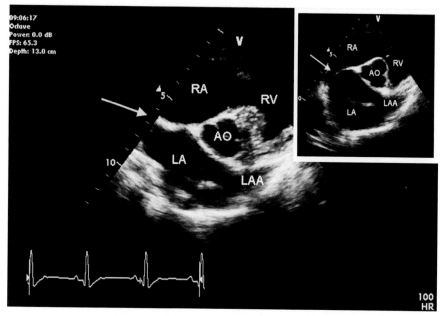

Figure 4.12 Over-rotated left atrium aorta view. When the interatrial septum is straight and located at about 9 o'clock on the sector image (arrow), the transducer has been over-rotated towards the sternum. Rotate the reference mark back towards the animal's elbows slightly until the atrial septum is slightly curved and directed downwards on the sector image. The inset shows an appropriate left atrium and interatrial septum (arrow) in the same dog. Note how over-rotation changes the size of the left atrium.

☐ Rotate the transducer back towards the animal's elbows until the interatrial septum is slightly curved and directed downward

LEFT PARASTERNAL IMAGING PLANES: CRANIAL LONG-AXIS VIEWS

Left Ventricular Outflow

Video 4.5

- Technique in the Dog and Cat (see Figure 4.13 and Video 4.5)
  - ○ Reference mark towards the front legs
  - ○ Crystals directed towards the shoulder blades
  - ○ Angle of about 45° between the transducer and the chest wall
  - ○ Place the transducer as far cranial and dorsal as possible to obtain this image
    - ■ Often you will feel the animal's triceps against your hand
  - ○ Slide within the two intercostal spaces behind the leg in a search mode from the costochondral junction to the sternum until the heart is seen

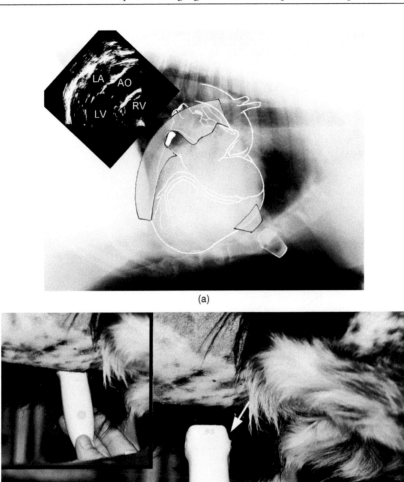

(a)

(b)

Figure 4.13 Radiographic plane and echocardiographic image of the left cranial long axis inflow outflow view. (a) The transducer is under the dog on the left side of the thorax, with the dog placed in left lateral recumbency over a hole in the scan table. The transducer is positioned in front of the heart pointing slightly back at it, as shown here. The sheet of sound is oriented along the length of the heart through the aorta. The corresponding echocardiographic imaging plane is shown to the top left in the same orientation as the sound plane through the thorax. **Transducer position for the left parasternal long-axis inflow outflow view.** (b) The transducer is placed on the left side of the thorax, in front of the heart. The reference mark is directed towards the heart base towards the front legs (arrow). The crystals (the surface of the transducer) are pointed at the shoulder blades, and there should be an angle of about 45° between the transducer and the chest wall. The smaller inset shows the transducer in position on the chest wall. It is located cranially and dorsally under this dog.

○ Lift the transducer up and down (making the angle between the transducer and the thorax larger and smaller but still pointing at the shoulder blades with the crystals) until an aorta is seen

○ Twist the transducer clockwise and counterclockwise until the aorta is as long as possible

Right Atrium and Auricle

• Technique in the dog and cat (see Figure 4.13(b), Figure 4.14 and Video 4.5)

○ Start with a good long-axis left ventricular outflow view

○ Make sure the aorta is as long as possible

▪ The longer and more horizontally oriented the long-axis aorta, the better the right auricular image will be

○ Drop the cable making the angle between the transducer and the thorax larger until the auricle comes into view

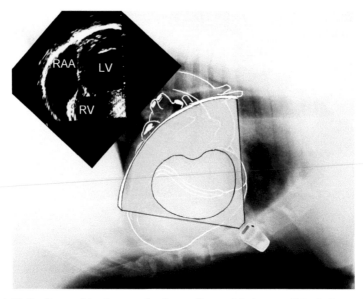

Figure 4.14 Radiographic plane and echocardiographic image of the left cranial long-axis right auricular view. The transducer is positioned in front of the heart, pointing back at it as shown here. The sheet of sound is oriented along the length of the heart but is directed upwards to the top of the heart. The angle between the transducer and the thorax has been increased to make this happen. The corresponding echocardiographic imaging plane is shown to the top left in the same orientation as the sound plane through the thorax.

Right Ventricular Outflow (Pulmonary Artery)

- Technique in the dog and cat (see Figure 4.13(b), Figure 4.15 and Video 4.5)
    - Start with a good long-axis left ventricular outflow view
    - Make sure the aorta is as long and horizontally oriented as possible
    - Lift the transducer making the angle between the transducer and the thorax smaller until the pulmonary artery comes into view

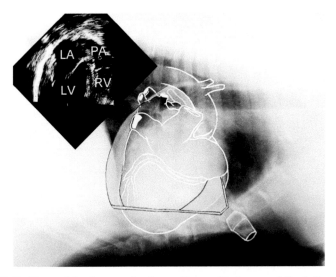

Figure 4.15 Radiographic plane and echocardiographic image of the left cranial long-axis pulmonary view. The transducer is under the dog on the left side of the thorax, with the dog placed in left lateral recumbency over a hole in the scan table. The transducer is positioned in front of the heart, pointing back at it as shown here. The sheet of sound is oriented along the length of the heart but is directed downward to the bottom of the heart. The angle between the transducer and the thorax has been decreased to make this happen. The corresponding echocardiographic imaging plane is shown to the top left in the same orientation as the sound plane through the thorax.

LEFT PARASTERNAL IMAGING PLANES: TRANSVERSE VIEWS

Transverse Heart Base

- Technique in the dog and cat (see Figure 4.16 and Video 4.5)
    - From the cranial long inflow outflow view
    - Twist the transducer so that the reference mark is directed towards the spine and down

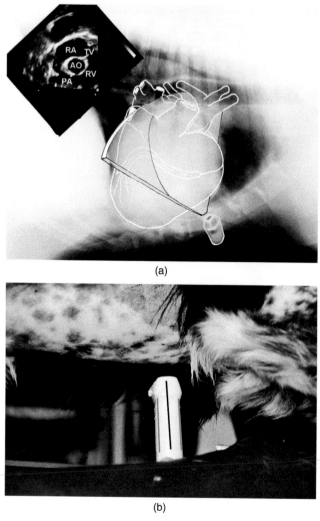

(a)

(b)

Figure 4.16 Radiographic plane and echocardiographic image of the left cranial short-axis view. (a) The transducer is under the dog on the left side of the thorax, with the dog placed in left lateral recumbency over a hole in the scan table. The sheet of sound is oriented along the short-axis plane of the heart. The transducer is in the same location as it was for the left cranial long-axis views. The corresponding echocardiographic imaging plane is shown to the top left in the same orientation as the sound plane through the thorax.
Transducer position for the left parasternal short-axis views of the heart. (b) The transducer is placed on the left side of the thorax, cranial and dorsal under the heart. The reference mark is directed towards the spine and downward opposite the black line on this transducer. There should be an angle of about 45° between the transducer and the chest wall.

- Twist until the aorta is seen as a circle in the transverse plane
- Fanning towards the heart base (front legs) with the crystals will bring in the pulmonary artery and fanning caudally (tail) should bring in the tricuspid valve and right atrium
  - It is often difficult to see both good tricuspid valve motion and the pulmonary artery at the same time – fanning between the two may be necessary

Left Auricle

Videos 4.5 and 4.6

- Technique in the cat (see Video 4.5 and Video 4.6)
  - From the cranial transverse view of the aorta described above
  - Between the plane of the pulmonary artery and the right atrium
    - The left auricle is seen to the right of the aorta as the crystals are fanned from the pulmonary artery caudally (to the tail)

LEFT PARASTERNAL IMAGING PLANES: APICAL VIEWS

Apical Four-Chamber

- Technique in the dog (see Figure 4.17 and Video 4.7)
  - Reference mark directed toward the spine and slightly down away from the dog's body
  - Point the crystals toward the neck (at the heart base)
  - About 30° between chest wall and transducer
  - Imagine the transducer as an extension of the length of the heart from base to apex
  - Find the liver near the last intercostal space, close to the sternum
  - Stay next to the sternum and slide cranial until the first intercostal space that the liver disappears and the beating heart is seen
    - The heart will typically not look good right here
  - Lift the transducer up towards the chest wall to bring in the heart base at the bottom of the sector image
  - Keep the crystals pointing toward the heart base
  - To perfect the image:
    - If the ventricle is not long (Figure 4.18)
      - Slide caudal and ventral keeping the angle between the transducer and thorax small (see Video 4.7)
      - The left ventricular chamber should be about twice as long as it is wide in the normal heart
    - The heart is not vertical on the image (Figure 4.19 and Video 4.7)

Video 4.7

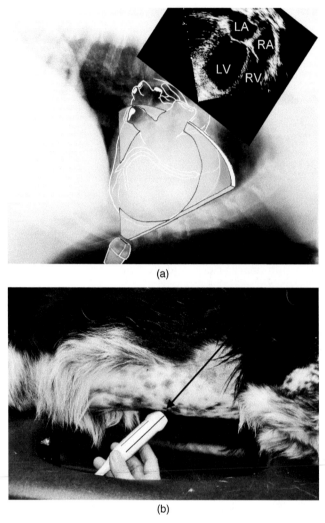

(a)

(b)

Figure 4.17 Radiographic plane and echocardiographic image of the left apical four-chamber view. (a) The transducer is under the dog on the left side of the thorax, with the dog placed in left lateral recumbency over a hole in the scan table. The transducer is positioned at the apex of the heart near the sternum, as shown here. The sheet of sound is directed along the length of the heart from apex to base so that the crystals are pointing at the heart base (shoulder blades). The corresponding echocardiographic imaging plane is shown to the top right in the same orientation as the sound plane through the thorax. **Transducer position for the left parasternal apical views of the heart.** (b) The transducer is placed on the left side of the thorax at the apex of the heart, near the sternum. The reference mark is directed towards the spine and slightly downward opposite the thick black line on this transducer. There should be an angle of about 45° between the transducer and the chest wall. The crystals are pointing towards the heart base (arrow).

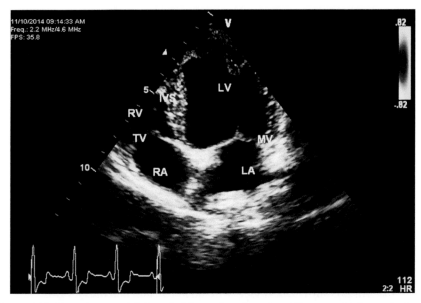

Figure 4.18 Foreshortened left apical four-chamber view. The normal left ventricular chamber should be about twice as long as it is wide. Here, the left ventricular chamber is short, being just slightly longer than it is wide. Since the apex is up at the top of the sector, simply sliding caudal and ventral (towards the apex) without changing where the crystals are pointed will elongate this heart. (See Video 4.7 and text for details.)

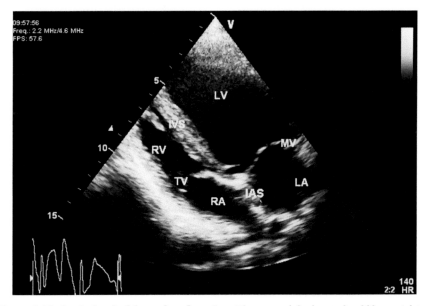

Figure 4.19 Angled apical four-chamber view. The apex of the heart should be upright enough, with the apex near the top of the sector and the base at the bottom in order to eventually line up Doppler cursors with flow through the aorta and mitral valve. Here, the heart is oriented more horizontally on the sector. Slide caudal and ventral towards the apex of the heart and then point the crystals more toward the heart base near the top of the shoulder blades. (See Video 4.7 and text for more details.)

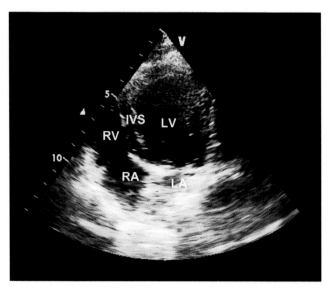

Figure 4.20 Apical four-chamber view with no left atrium and mitral valve. This apical four-chamber view of the heart does not have a clear left atrium, and the mitral valve would not be moving if this were a video. The transducer needs to be rotated so that the reference mark moves down away from the thorax in order to fix this problem. (See Video 4.7 and text for more details).

- □ A Doppler cursor should align with the walls of the aorta and mitral valve flow
- □ Fan not rotate the transducer crystals in a ventral or dorsal direction to straighten up the apical view
- □ Usually, once the apex is located at the top of the sector, the transducer needs to be moved toward the sternum and maybe caudal one intercostal space to lengthen the heart
- The mitral valve and left atrium are not seen well in the four-chamber view (Figure 4.20)
  - □ Rotate the reference mark down away from the thorax until the left atrium is seen and the mitral valve moves well
  - □ Adjust the angle between the transducer and the thorax to optimize the four-chamber view
- Technique in the cat
  - ○ The difference between a cat and dog is in how the heart is oriented in the thorax (see Figures 4.21 and 1.4)
  - ○ Feline hearts are oriented more in line with the sternum, so the transducer crystals will point more towards the front legs instead of the shoulder blades

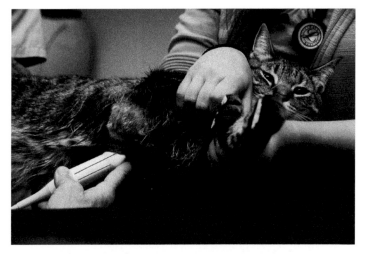

Figure 4.21 Transducer position for the left parasternal apical views of the heart in the cat. The transducer is placed on the left side of the thorax at the apex of the heart, near the sternum. The reference mark is directed towards the spine and slightly downward opposite the thick black line on this transducer. There should be an angle of about 45° or less between the transducer and the chest wall. The crystals are pointing towards the heart base, which is less toward the shoulder blades, and more towards the front legs. In the cat the transducer is aligned more parallel with the body since the feline heart is oriented more along the sternum.

- ○ Reference mark directed towards the spine and slightly down away from the cat's thorax
- ○ Point the crystals toward the front legs (heart base)
- ○ Small angle between chest wall and transducer of about 20–30°
  - ■ The transducer hugs the abdominal wall in some cats
- ○ Find the liver near the last intercostal space, close to the sternum
- ○ Stay next to the sternum and slide forward until the liver disappears and the heart is seen
  - ■ The heart will typically not look good right here
- ○ Lift the transducer up towards the chest wall to bring in the heart base
- ○ If the ventricle is not long, slide caudal and ventral and keep the angle between the transducer and thorax small

Apical Five-Chamber

- Technique in the dog and cat (see Figure 4.22 and Video 4.7)
  - ○ Start with a good apical four-chamber view
  - ○ Lift the transducer even more towards the chest wall making the angle between the transducer and the thorax smaller

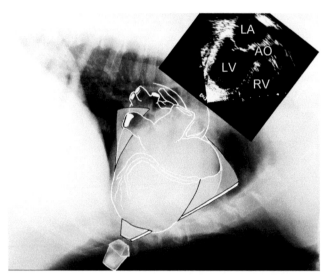

Figure 4.22 Radiographic plane and echocardiographic image of the left apical five-chamber view. The transducer is under the dog on the left side of the thorax, with the dog placed in left lateral recumbency over a hole in the scan table. The transducer is positioned at the apex of the heart near the sternum, as shown here. The sheet of sound is directed along the length of the heart from apex to base, so that the crystals are pointing at the heart base (shoulder blades). The transducer has a smaller angle between it and the chest wall than what is present in the four-chamber view. The corresponding echocardiographic imaging plane is shown to the top right in the same orientation as the sound plane through the thorax.

- The transducer may be very parallel with the scan table at this point, especially in cats
  ○ Rotate the reference mark down or up slightly if necessary to see the aorta well

Chapter 5 M-Mode Echocardiography

Principles of M-Mode Echocardiography

- One single sound beam is selected over the real time image
  - Select a location with the cursor and track ball
- The structures under the cursor are seen on the M-mode image (Figure 5.1 and Video 5.1)
- The M-mode diagram has depth on the y-axis and time on the x-axis
- The M-mode scrolls across the screen showing the cardiac structures as they change during diastole and systole
- Freeze the desired M-mode for measuring
  - The image should have clearly defined structural boundaries

Video 5.1

M-Mode of the Left Ventricle

- The cursor may be placed over right parasternal long- or short-axis images
- Using the long axis
  - Use the right parasternal left ventricular outflow view (inflow outflow view)
    - It should be optimized for length and width, a clear aorta and aortic valve, well-moving mitral valve
      - □ The wall and the septum are parallel to each other when the left ventricular size is optimized

Two-Dimensional and M-Mode Echocardiography for the Small Animal Practitioner, Second Edition. June A. Boon.
© 2017 John Wiley & Sons, Inc. Published 2017 by John Wiley & Sons, Inc.
Companion Website: www.wiley.com/go/boon/two-dimensional

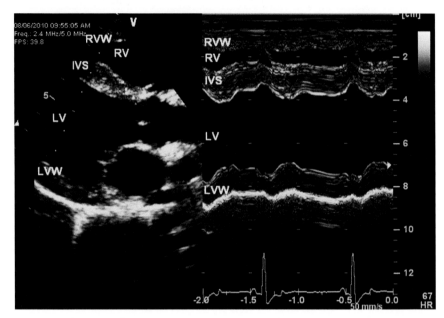

Figure 5.1 The M-mode image. M-mode images show the structures under a line placed over the two-dimensional image. Here, the line is placed over the left ventricle on a long-axis inflow outflow view. The M-mode shows the same cardiac structures from the top of the sector image to the bottom, as are seen on the two-dimensional inflow outflow view. The y-axis represents centimeters of depth, and the x-axis is time. The same place in the heart is displayed over time on the x-axis as the structures change and move during systole and diastole. For details of abbreviations used in the figures, see the Glossary.

Video 5.2

- ■ Place the cursor perpendicular to the septum and free wall at the largest ventricular dimension between the tips of the mitral valve leaflets and the papillary muscles (see Figures 5.1 and 5.2 and Videos 5.1 and 5.2)
- ■ Make sure you are not placing the cursor over the thinner part of the septum within the left ventricular outflow tract (see Figure 5.2)
- • Using the short axis
  - ○ Use the right parasternal transverse view at the level of the chordae tendineae

Video 5.3

  - ■ Fan the sound beam between the mitral valve and papillary muscles in order to find the level of the chordae (see Figure 5.3 and Video 5.3)
    - ▢ The image should be symmetrical
    - ▢ It should be the smallest transverse plane at the level of the chordae
    - ▢ There should be a good right ventricular chamber above the left ventricular chamber
    - ▢ The lack of a right ventricular chamber means the transducer is placed too close to the apex of the heart
  - ■ Place the cursor through the middle of the left ventricular chamber making two similar halves that are mirror images of each other (Figure 5.3 and Video 5.3)

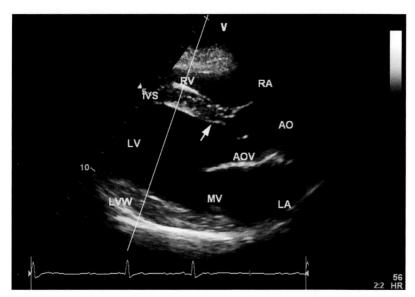

Figure 5.2 Cursor placement: Left ventricular M-mode from the long axis. Use the right parasternal long-axis image left ventricular inflow outflow view that is optimized for length and width, has a clear aorta and aortic valve, and well-moving mitral valve leaflets (see text for details). Place the cursor perpendicular to the septum and left ventricular wall at the largest ventricular dimension between the tips of the mitral valve leaflets and the papillary muscles. The papillary muscles should not be visible during diastole, as this image shows. Do not place the cursor over the thinner less contractile area at the base of the interventricular septum (arrow). (See Video 5.1.)

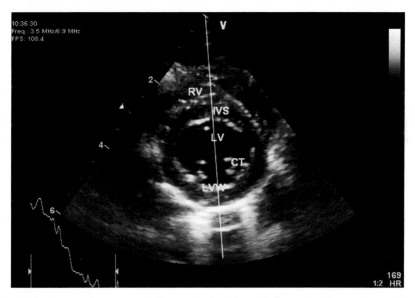

Figure 5.3 Cursor placement: Left ventricular M-mode from the short axis. Fan the sound beam between the transverse image of the mitral valve leaflets and the papillary muscles in order to find the smallest symmetrical chamber at the level of the chordae. Place the cursor through the middle of the left ventricular chamber, making two similar halves – these will be mirror images of each other.

- The Left Ventricular M-mode Image
  - Structures from the top of the two-dimensional image to the bottom of the sector are displayed in the same order from top to bottom on the M-mode image (see Figure 5.1).
  - The interventricular septum and left ventricular wall become thicker during systole and thinner during diastole (Figure 5.1 and Video 5.3)
  - The left ventricular chamber becomes larger during diastole and smaller during systole (Figure 5.1 and Video 5.3)

M-Mode of the Aorta and Left Atrium

- These images may be obtained from right parasternal long- or short-axis images
- Using the long-axis images
  - Use the left ventricular inflow outflow view optimized for length and width (see Figures 5.2 and 5.4 and Videos 5.2 and 5.4)

Video 5.4

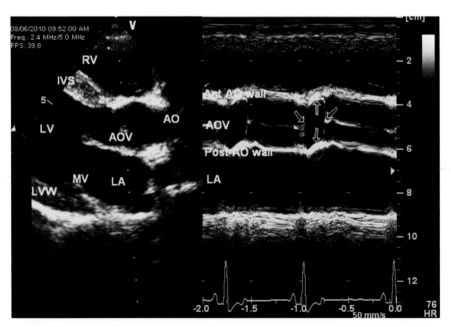

Figure 5.4 Cursor placement: Aorta left atrium M-mode from the long axis. Use an inflow outflow view optimized for length and width (see text for details). Place the cursor perpendicular to the walls of the aorta over the valve cusps. This should place the cursor automatically through the largest portion of the left atrium. The walls of the aorta will be represented by two parallel lines, the aortic valve is seen between these walls. The aortic valve is a line in the middle of the aorta during diastole and opens into a box shape during systole. Arrows show where the aortic valve opens and closes, and its excursion to the anterior and posterior walls.

- Place the cursor perpendicular to the walls of the aorta over the aortic valve cusps
- The cusps themselves are not always visualized well, but the dash that represents cusp coaptation should be in the middle of the aorta
- This should place the cursor automatically through the largest portion of the left atrium
- The left ventricular chamber should be as long and wide as possible (see Figure 5.2)
  - The wall and the septum should be parallel to each other if the chamber is as long as it can be
- The mitral valve should move well and be clearly seen
- Sometimes you must slide the image to the left side of the sector to align the cursor properly
- Using the short axis
  - Use the transverse heart base view with all three aortic valve cusps visible (Figure 5.5 and Video 5.5)
    - Place the cursor through the middle of the aorta through or close to the line that defines the junction of the non and left coronary cusps
    - The aorta is a closed circle with the "Mercedes" sign visible

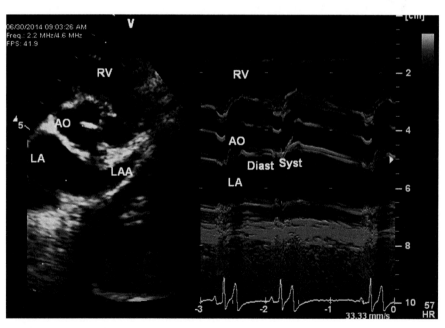

Figure 5.5 Cursor placement: Aorta left atrium M-mode from the short axis. Place the cursor through the centre of the aorta through the aortic valve on the right parasternal transverse view. The three aortic valve cusps and the left atrium and auricle are clearly seen. Make sure the cursor is not in the left auricular appendage, but is to the left of it in the left atrial chamber. The cursor should be through or close to the line that defines the junction of the non and left coronary cusps.

- The left atrium and auricle are clearly seen
- Do not have the pulmonary artery in the image
  - The cursor should be aligned through the left atrium, not the auricle
  - The image may have to be oriented towards the left side of the monitor for this to work
- The Aorta and Left Atrium M-mode image
  - The aorta is two parallel lines, the anterior aortic wall and the posterior aortic wall (see Figures 5.4 and 5.5 and Videos 5.4 and 5.5)
  - The line in the middle of the aorta is the aortic valve during diastole, and these cusps open to the anterior and posterior wall during systole, creating a box shape while open.
  - The left atrium is below the aorta, and fills during systole when the mitral valve is closed and the aortic valve is open.
  - Structures from the top of the two-dimensional image to the bottom of the sector are displayed in the same order from top to bottom on the M-mode image

M-Mode of the Mitral Valve

- This image may be made from either the right parasternal long- or short-axis views
- From the long axis
  - Use the left ventricular outflow view (inflow outflow view)
    - Make sure the mitral valve moves well and that the aortic valve is also seen
      - The aortic valve cusps may not be clearly seen but the dash in the middle of the aorta representing the closed valve should be seen

Video 5.6

    - Place the cursor over the tips of the mitral valve leaflets (Figure 5.6 and Video 5.6)
    - The cursor should be fairly perpendicular to the septum, and not diagonal through the left ventricular chamber
- From the short axis
  - Use the transverse view where both leaflets are seen (the "fish mouth" view)
    - Make the image symmetrical
    - Place the cursor through the middle of the chamber through the middle of the mitral valve leaflets
- The Mitral Valve M-mode Image
  - At slower heart rates the anterior leaflet of the mitral valve should have an "M" configuration, while the posterior leaflet should have a "W" shape (see Figures 5.6 and 5.7 and Videos 5.6 and 5.7)

Video 5.7

  - The first peak of the M represents rapid ventricular filling and is called the "E" point or peak for rapid early diastolic filling

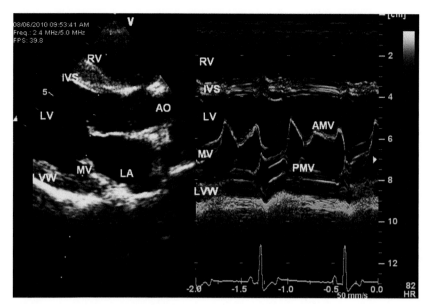

Figure 5.6 Cursor placement: Mitral valve M-mode from the long axis. Using a right parasternal long-axis inflow outflow view optimized for length and width (see text for details), place the cursor relatively perpendicular to the septum and left ventricular wall at the tips of the mitral valve leaflets.

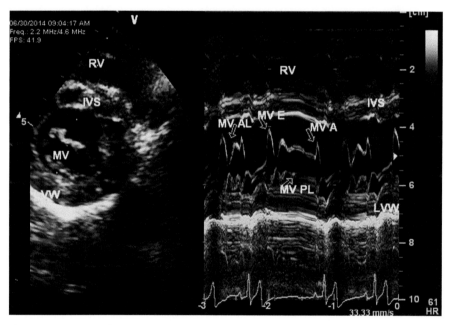

Figure 5.7 Cursor placement: Mitral valve M-mode from the short axis. Use the right parasternal transverse view of the mitral valve where both leaflets are seen (the "fish mouth" view). Make the image symmetrical and place the cursor through the middle of the chamber and fish mouth. Structures from the top of the two-dimensional image to the bottom of the sector are displayed in the same order from top to bottom on the M-mode image. Early diastolic filling results in a rapid upward motion of the mitral valve called the E peak, while the atrial contraction at the end of diastole results in an upward motion called the A peak.

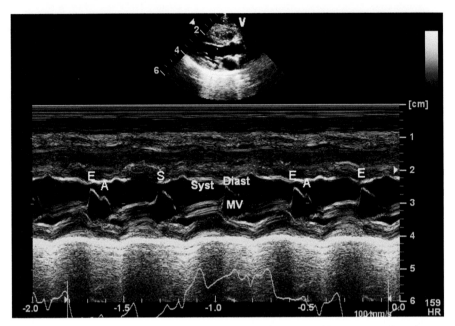

Figure 5.8 Summation of mitral valve E and A peaks. At rapid heart rates, when the diastolic time period becomes shorter, the two phases of filling begin to overlap until at some point the filling period is so short that only one component of filling is appreciated on the M-mode image. This results in summated E and A waves. The single peak is referred to as the E peak. In this cat, mitral valve summation (S) is indicated by the single E waves.

- The atrium has been filling throughout ventricular systole; at the beginning of diastole the pressure gradient from the left atrium to the left ventricle causes the anterior mitral valve to passively, but rapidly, open up towards the septum creating the E peak. The posterior leaflet moves downward towards the left ventricular wall
- After the initial filling phase the pressures equilibrate somewhat and the flow decreases
  - The mitral valve moves towards a partially closed position
- Atrial contraction towards the end of diastole causes the anterior mitral valve leaflet to actively open towards the septum, and the posterior mitral valve leaflet to move downwards to the free wall again
- This creates the second peak of the "M" and is referred to as the "A" point or peak for the atrial contraction
  - At rapid heart rates, when the diastolic time period becomes shorter, the two phases of filling begin to overlap until at some point the filling period is so short that only one component of filling is appreciated on the M-mode image. This results in summated E and A waves (Figure 5.8)

Chapter 6 Measurement and Assessment of Two-Dimensional and M-Mode Images

Measurement of the Left Ventricular Chamber

- Diastolic measurements – Timing
  - These should be made at the onset of the QRS complex if you have an ECG on both two-dimensional and M-mode images
  - Without an ECG, measure at the largest left ventricular dimension on the two-dimensional image and just before the wall and septum begin to thicken on M-mode images (Figures 6.1 and 6.2)
- Systolic Measurements – Timing
  - These are made at the smallest left ventricular chamber size on both two-dimensional and M-mode images (see Figures 6.1, 6.2 and 6.3)
  - When the septum and the wall do not peak at the same time in systole, measure the smallest chamber size (see Figure 6.2(a)). If the wall and septum are very dys-synchronous (see Figure 6.2(b)) measure the left ventricle on two-dimensional images

---

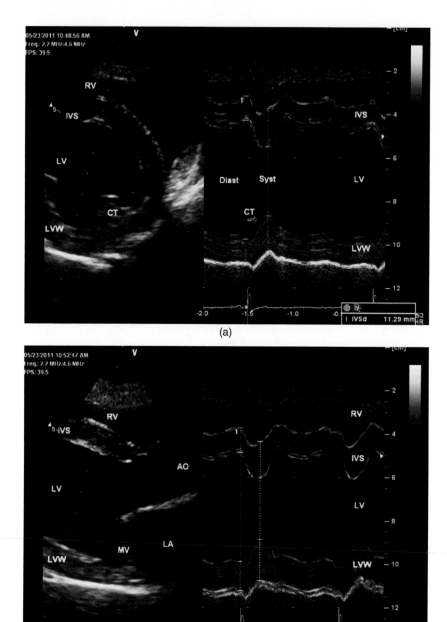

Figure 6.1 M-mode left ventricular measurements. (a, b) Make diastolic measurements at the beginning of the QRS complex or at the largest chamber size. Make systolic measurements at the smallest chamber size. The measurements are made at the same places on the M-mode whether the M-mode is obtained from short-axis (a) or long-axis (b views. The dashes and dotted lines show where measurements are made. The interventricular septum is measured from the top of the septum to the bottom of the septum, the left ventricular chamber from the bottom of the septum to the top of the left ventricular wall, and the left ventricular wall from the top of the wall to the top of the pericardial sac. For details of abbreviations used in the figures, see the Glossary.

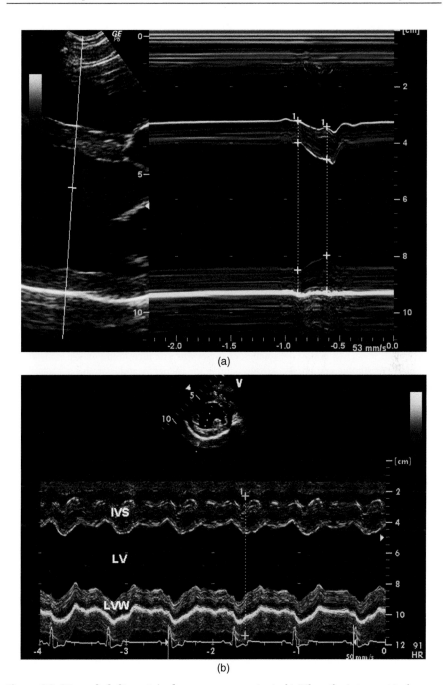

(a)

(b)

Figure 6.2 M-mode left ventricular measurements. (a, b) When the interventricular septum and left ventricular wall do not peak at the same time during systole, measure the smallest chamber size (a) unless they are significantly dys-synchronous (b). You should then measure on two-dimensional images as the measurements of left ventricular size and function will not be accurate using the m-mode.

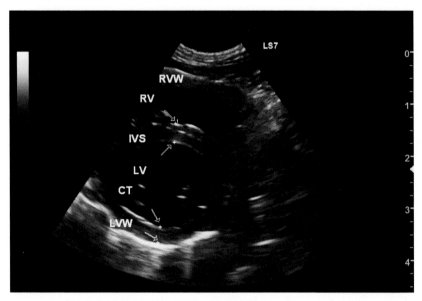

Figure 6.3 Two-dimensional left ventricular measurements. Make diastolic measurements at the beginning of the QRS complex if present, or at the largest chamber size. Make systolic measurements at the smallest chamber size. The measurements are made at the same places in diastole and systole. Arrows point at the caliper locations on this diastolic transverse left ventricular chamber at the level of the chordae. The interventricular septum is measured from the top of the septum to the bottom of the septum, the left ventricular chamber from the bottom of the septum to the top of the left ventricular wall, and the left ventricular wall from the top of the wall to the top of the pericardial sac.

- Location
  - Measure both diastolic and systolic parameters in the following manner on M-mode images and on two-dimensional images (see Figures 6.1, 6.2 and 6.3):
    - Interventricular septum – from above the line that defines the top of the septum to on top of the line that defines the bottom of the septum
    - Left ventricular chamber – from on top of the line that defines the bottom of the septum to the top of the line that defines the left ventricular wall
    - Left ventricular wall – from the top of the line that defines the top of the wall to the top f the pericardial sac (see Figures 6.1, 6.2 and 6.3)

Measurement of the Aorta and Left Atrium

- M-mode measurements
  - Aorta – measured at end-diastole
    - These measurements are made at the onset of the QRS complex

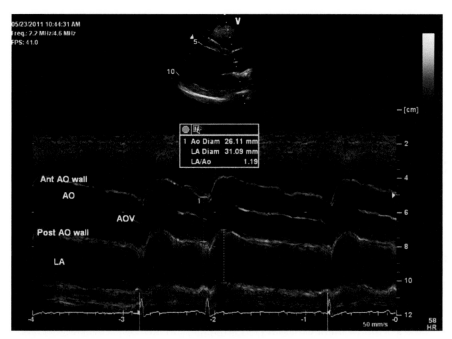

Figure 6.4 M-mode aorta left atrium measurements. The aorta is measured at end-diastole with the beginning of the QRS complex, or just before the aortic valve opens if an ECG is not available. Left atrial size is measured at its largest dimension at the end of systole. Measure from the top of the line that defines the anterior (top) aortic wall to the top of the line that defines the posterior (bottom) aortic wall. The left atrium is measured at about end-systole at the largest left atrial chamber size, when the posterior aortic wall is at its highest point. Measure from the top of line that defines the posterior aortic wall to the top of the pericardium. Dashes and dotted lines show caliper locations. See text for more details.

- If an ECG is not available, measure at the lowest point of aortic wall motion just before the aortic valve opens (Figure 6.4)
- Measure from the top of the line that defines the anterior (top) aortic wall to the top of the line that defines the posterior (bottom) aortic wall
- The line representing the top of the aorta is included in the measurement but the bottom line is not
  - Left atrium – measured at about end-systole (see Figure 6.4)
    - These measurements are made at the largest left atrial chamber size when the posterior aortic wall is at its highest point
    - Measure from the top of the line that defines the posterior aortic wall to the top of the pericardium
    - The line representing the bottom of the aorta is included in this atrial measurement, whereas it is not included in the aortic measurement
    - If a left atrial wall is seen, ignore it and measure down to the top of the pericardium

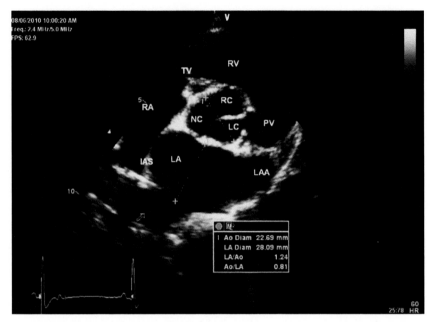

Figure 6.5 Rishniw method of aorta left atrial measurement. On a transverse view of the aorta and left atrium at the first frame just after aortic valve closure before the left atrium starts to become smaller, measure the aorta and left atrium. Measure the internal dimension of the aorta along the line that defines the border of the right and noncoronary cusps. Measure the internal dimension of the left atrium in a direction that extends the line defining the border of the noncoronary and left coronary cusps. Calipers and dotted lines show measurement locations. The arrow is pointing at a pulmonary vein; measure to a place that is perceived to be where the atrial wall would be.

- Two-dimensional measurements
    - Rishniw method – use the short-axis aorta left atrium image (see Figure 6.5)
        - These measurements are made at the first frame after the aortic valve closes
        - Measure the internal dimension of the aorta along the line that defines the border of the right and noncoronary cusps
        - Measure the internal dimension of the left atrium in a direction that extends the line defining the border of the noncoronary and left coronary cusps
        - If a pulmonary vein is seen, then the atrial wall is extrapolated and the atrial measurement is stopped at the perceived wall location.
    - Swedish Method – use the short-axis aorta left atrium image (see Figure 6.6)
        - These measurements are made at the first frame after the aortic valve closes
        - Measure from the top of the line that defines the wall of the aorta to the top of the line that defines the bottom of the aorta along the line defined by the junction of the noncoronary and left coronary cusps

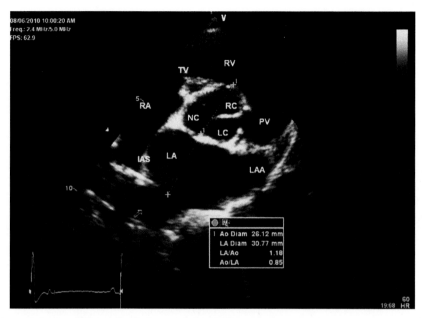

Figure 6.6 Swedish method of aorta left atrial measurement. On a transverse view of the aorta and left atrium, at the frame just after aortic valve closure before the left atrium starts to become smaller. Include the anterior aortic wall in the aortic measurement and the posterior aortic wall in the left atrial measurement. Calipers and dotted lines show measurement locations. The arrow is pointing at a pulmonary vein; measure to a place that is perceived to be where the atrial wall would be (see text for details).

- ■ Measure from the top of the line that defines the aortic wall through the left atrium in a direction that extends the line defining the border of the noncoronary and left coronary cusps
- ■ If a pulmonary vein is seen, then the atrial wall is extrapolated and the atrial measurement is stopped at the perceived wall location.

Measurement of the Mitral Valve

- • M-mode images
  - ○ Typically only measured on M-mode images
  - ○ The only consistent measurement for the mitral valve is the E peak to septal separation (EPSS)
    - ■ Measure from the top of the E peak to the bottom of the septum (see Figure 6.7)
    - ■ The EPSS is measured from the single peak in summated E and A waves
    - ■ Do not include the line defining the bottom of the septum in the measurement

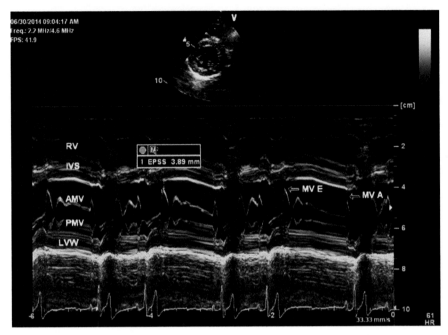

Figure 6.7 Measurement of the mitral valve – EPSS. The E peak to septal separation (EPSS) is measured from the top of the E peak to the bottom of the interventricular septum. (see text for details).

Assessment of Two-Dimensional and M-Mode Measurements

- Left ventricular size
  - Measurements of chamber size and wall thicknesses should be similar whether obtained from long-axis or short-axis views or from M-mode or two-dimensional images when done correctly
    - Diastolic measurements
      - Used to assess chamber sizes (see Figures 6.8–6.11)
        - Larger diastolic measurements reflect increased volume within that chamber
        - Smaller measurements reflect reduced volumes
      - Used to assess left ventricular wall and septal thicknesses (see Figures 6.8–6.11)
        - Increased diastolic wall or septal measurements reflect hypertrophy or pseudohypertrophy secondary to poor preload (see below)
        - Thinning of the wall or septum is reflected in smaller than expected diastolic measurements

Echocardiographic Measurements

		95%	CI
Septum - d (mm)	13.2	11.5	13.4
LV chamber - d (mm)	56.3	40.6	42.5
LV wall - d (mm)	10.1	9.3	10.9
Septum - s (mm)	18.0	17.7	19.8
LV chamber - s (mm)	25.2	25.6	27.3
LV wall - s (mm)	16.1	15.0	16.9
Fractional shortening (%)	55.2	30.0	46.0

Figure 6.8 Assessment of left ventricular size and function. Diastolic measurements are used to determine if the left ventricle is dilated, normal or small, and to decide if the wall and septum are hypertrophied, normal or thin. Here, the left ventricular chamber is dilated and the wall and septum are normal in thickness. Systolic chamber size reflects function of the heart. Here, a normal systolic chamber size is consistent with normal contractility. The elevated fractional shortening reflects elevated function, which should be expected if myocardial contractility is preserved since the dilation puts more stretch on the myofibers.

Echocardiographic Measurements

		95%	CI
Septum - d (mm)	16.1	11.5	13.4
LV chamber - d (mm)	36.1	40.6	42.5
LV wall - d (mm)	15.5	9.3	10.9
Septum - s (mm)	21.0	17.7	19.8
LV chamber - s (mm)	29.1	25.6	27.3
LV wall - s (mm)	17.2	15.0	16.9
Fractional shortening (%)	19.4	30.0	46.0

Figure 6.9 Assessment of left ventricular size and function. Diastolic measurements are used to determine if the left ventricle is dilated, normal or small, and to decide if the wall and septum are hypertrophied, normal or thin. Here, the left ventricular chamber is small and the wall and septum are thicker than expected. These abnormalities are seen with left ventricular hypertrophy or decreased preload (pseudohypertrophy). The slightly increased systolic chamber size and depressed fractional shortening are consistent with poor function, and may be normal variation or a reflection of poor contractility or secondary to elevated afterload.

Echocardiographic Measurements

		95%	CI
Septum - d (mm)	9.0	11.5	13.4
LV chamber - d (mm)	56.3	40.6	42.5
LV wall - d (mm)	8.1	9.3	10.9
Septum - s (mm)	16.0	17.7	19.8
LV chamber - s (mm)	39.1	25.6	27.3
LV wall - s (mm)	13.5	15.0	16.9
Fractional shortening (%)	30.6	30.0	46.0

Figure 6.10 Assessment of left ventricular size and function. Diastolic measurements are used to determine if the left ventricle is dilated, normal or small, and to decide if the wall and septum are hypertrophied, normal or thin. Here, the left ventricular chamber is dilated and the wall and septum are thin. The systolic left ventricular chamber is large, consistent with either poor contractility or high afterload. If blood pressure is normal, then contractility is depressed. If blood pressure is elevated, then the large systolic dimension may be secondary to the muscle's inability to shorten against that load. Contractility cannot be accurately assessed until the blood pressure is normalized. Fractional shortening is normal and is a misleading number here.

Echocardiographic Measurements

		95%	CI
Septum - d (mm)	9.4	9.6	10.6
LV chamber - d (mm)	36.0	35.3	36.7
LV wall - d (mm)	7.9	7.8	8.6
Septum - s (mm)	16.5	14.6	15.6
LV chamber - s (mm)	22.0	22.0	23.2
LV wall - s (mm)	14.5	12.5	13.5
Fractional shortening (%)	38.9	30.0	46.0

Figure 6.11 Assessment of left ventricular size and function. Diastolic measurements are used to determine if the left ventricle is dilated, normal or small, and to decide if the wall and septum are hypertrophied, normal or thin. Here, the left ventricular chamber is normal and the wall and septum are normal thickness. Do not become overzealous in calling a fraction of a mm or a mm out of the normal range an abnormal finding, as is seen in this septal thickness in diastole.The increased systolic thickness of the left ventricular wall and septum reflects systolic function, not hypertrophy. A normal systolic chamber size reflects normal function and contractility.

- Systolic measurements
  - Used to assess function (see Figures 6.8–6.11)
    - Increased left ventricular wall or septal thicknesses during systole reflect elevated function and not hypertrophy (although there may be hypertrophy which is assessed during diastole)
    - Increased systolic left ventricular chamber size reflects decreased function of the heart which may be secondary to poor contractility or increased blood pressure, not increased volume (although there may be an increased volume which is assessed during diastole)
- Types of ventricular enlargement
  - Left ventricular concentric hypertrophy
    - Increased septal and/or free wall thicknesses using diastolic numbers with a normal or small left ventricular chamber size (see Figure 6.9)
    - Causes of LV concentric hypertrophy
      - Hypertrophic cardiomyopathy
      - It may be secondary to increased workload (afterload) on the heart. Afterload is the work the ventricle must deal with during contraction, and includes the following causes:
        - Subaortic stenosis
        - Systemic hypertension
        - Lack of adequate hypertrophy for the volume in the heart
      - It may be "pseudo" hypertrophy
        - Volume contraction decreases chamber size and makes the walls appear thick when there is not as much stretch on the myofibers as there normally would be. This is called "poor preload," the load the ventricle must deal with before contraction.

- ◆ Causes of poor preload include:
  - ◇ Dehydration
  - ◇ Hemorrhage
  - ◇ Addison's disease
  - ◇ Moderate to severe pulmonic stenosis (decreased volume into the left heart)
  - ◇ Moderate to severe pulmonary hypertension (decreased volume into the left heart)
- ○ Right ventricular concentric hypertrophy:
  - ■ RV wall thickness greater than 1/2 of LV wall thickness in diastole
  - ■ Causes of RV concentric hypertrophy
    - ▫ Pulmonary stenosis
    - ▫ Pulmonary hypertension
    - ▫ Significant volume contraction
- ○ Left ventricular eccentric hypertrophy:
  - ■ Increased left ventricular chamber size, with or without measureable hypertrophy of the wall and septum. This is increased preload (see Figures 6.8, 6.10 and 6.11)
  - ■ Causes of LV eccentric hypertrophy
    - ▫ Valvular insufficiencies
      - ◆ Mitral
      - ◆ Aortic
    - ▫ Shunts
      - ◆ Patent ductus arteriosus (PDA)
      - ◆ Ventricular septal defect (VSD)
    - ▫ Miscellaneous
      - ◆ Chronic anemia
      - ◆ Systemic hypertension (later stages)
      - ◆ Dilated cardiomyopathy
- ○ Right ventricular eccentric hypertrophy:
  - ■ Increased chamber size – larger than 1/2 LV chamber size
  - ■ Causes of RV eccentric hypertrophy
    - ▫ Tricuspid regurgitation
    - ▫ Severe pulmonary insufficiency
    - ▫ Acute or acute on chronic pulmonary hypertension
- Left ventricular function (fractional shortening)
  - ○ This is an index of overall cardiac function
  - ○ It is the percentage change in left ventricular dimension between diastole and systole
  - ○ Many factors affect it, but the following are important to consider (see Figures 6.8–6.11):
    - ■ Preload
      - ▫ Increased preload (increased left ventricular chamber size) increases fractional shortening if contractility is normal

- ◆ Increased preload stretches the myocardial fibers, allowing the muscle fibers to slide over each other to a greater extent (Frank–Starling effect) and fiber shortening increases
  - □ Decreased preload (small left ventricular chamber size) decreases fractional shortening
    - ◆ Decreased preload decreases the amount of stretch on the muscle fibers, diminishing their ability to slide over each other, so that fiber shortening is decreased
- ■ Afterload
  - □ Increased afterload (blood pressure or inadequate hypertrophic responses) decreases fractional shortening
    - ◆ Increased afterload without chronicity diminishes the ability to shorten myofibers (think of pressing a free weight you are not used to), even if the muscle is normal
  - □ Decreased afterload increases fractional shortening
    - ◆ A lower blood pressure makes it easier for the muscle to contract, increasing fiber shortening
- ■ Contractility
  - □ Decreased contractility decreases fractional shortening
  - □ Increased contractility increases fractional shortening
  - □ A basic physiologic premise is that if contractility and afterload are normal, then the muscle will shorten to its normal systolic length; this means that the left ventricle will also shorten to is normal systolic chamber size, no matter what the preload status of the heart is.
- o A large systolic chamber size may be due to:
  - ■ Poor contractility
  - ■ High blood pressure (high afterload)
    - □ Without a blood pressure the final assessment of poor contractility cannot be made

Table 6.1 When contractility is normal, the following changes in preload and afterload affect fractional shortening (FS) as shown.

Condition	%FS
Preload	
Increased preload	↑
Decreased preload	↓
Afterload	
Increased afterload	↓
Decreased afterload	↑

Echocardiographic Reference Values

Table 6.2 Echocardiographic reference values for parameters of size in the cat.

Parameter	95% CI
Aorta (M-mode) (mm)	6.0–12.1
Left atrium (M-mode) (mm)	7.0–17.0
LA/AO	0.88–1.79
Interventricular septum – diastole (mm)	3.0–6.0
Left ventricle diameter – diastole (mm)	10.8–21.4
Left ventricular wall – diastole (mm)	2.5–6.0
Interventricular septum – systole (mm)	4.0–9.0
Left ventricle diameter – systole (mm)	4.0–11.2
Left ventricular wall – systole (mm)	4.3–9.8
Fractional shortening (%)	40–67
Left atrium (2D) (mm)	<14.5
LA/AO (2D)	<1.6

mm = millimeters; LA = left atrium; AO = aorta.
Data from:
Sisson, D., Helinski, C., et al. (1991) Plasma taurine concentrations and M-mode echocardiographic measures in healthy cats and cats with dilated cardiomyopathy. *J. Vet. Intern. Med.*, **5**, 232–238.
Jacobs, G. and Knight, D. (1985) M-mode echocardiographic measurements in non-anesthetized healthy cats: effects of body weight, heart rate, and other variables. *Am. J. Vet. Res.*, **46**, 1705–1711.
Abbott, J.A. and MacLean, H.N. (2006) Two-dimensional echocardiographic assessment of the feline left atrium. *J. Vet. Intern. Med.*, **20**, 111–119.

Table 6.3 Echocardiographic reference values for parameters of size in the Maine Coon cat.

Parameter	95% CI
Aorta (M-mode) (mm)	8.1–15.7
Left atrium (M-mode) (mm)	10.3–17.6
LA/AO	0.86–1.84
Interventricular septum – diastole (mm)	2.5–5.7
Left ventricle diameter – diastole (mm)	12.1–23.3
Left ventricular wall – diastole (mm)	2.8–5.9
Interventricular septum – systole (mm)	4.9–10.4
Left ventricle diameter – systole (mm)	5.0–14.5
Left ventricular wall – systole (mm)	5.4–10.7
Fractional shortening (%)	32–70

mm = millimeters; LA = left atrium; AO = aorta.
Data from:
Drourr, L., Lefbom, B.K., Rosenthal, S.L., et al. (2005) Measurement of M-mode echocardiographic parameters in healthy adult Maine Coon cats. *J. Am. Vet. Med. Assoc.*, **226**, 734–737.

Table 6.4 Echocardiographic reference values for parameters of size in the dog.

| | | CANINE M-MODE REFERENCE RANGES | | | | | | | |
| | | 95% prediction intervals (mm) | | | | | | | |
kg	Lbs	VSd	LVd	LVWd	VSs	LVs	LVWs	AO	LA
0.5	1	4.4–6.8	-7.7–4.2	3.5–5.4	6.7–9.4	-8.7–1.6	6.1–8.5	-11.3–2.6	-14.2–1.2
0.9	2	4.7–6.9	-1.2–10.7	3.7–5.5	7.1–9.6	-4.2–6.1	6.4–8.7	-6.7–7.2	-8.4–7.1
1.4	3	4.9–7.1	2.7–14.5	3.9–5.6	7.4–9.8	-1.5–8.8	6.7–8.9	-4.0–9.9	-5.0–10.5
1.8	4	5.1–7.2	5.4–17.2	4.0–5.7	7.7–10.0	0.3–10.7	6.9–9.1	-2.1–11.8	-2.6–12.9
2.3	5	5.3–7.3	7.5–19.3	4.2–5.8	7.9–10.2	1.8–12.1	7.1–9.2	-0.6–13.3	-0.7–14.8
2.7	6	5.4–7.4	9.2–21.0	4.3–5.9	8.2–10.3	3.0–13.3	7.3–9.3	0.6–14.5	0.9–16.3
3.2	7	5.6–7.4	10.7–22.5	4.4–6.0	8.4–10.5	4.0–14.3	7.5–9.4	1.7–15.5	2.2–17.6
3.6	8	5.7–7.5	11.9–23.7	4.5–6.0	8.6–10.6	4.9–15.2	7.7–9.6	2.6–16.4	3.3–18.7
4.1	9	5.8–7.6	13.0–24.8	4.6–6.1	8.8–10.8	5.6–15.9	7.8–9.7	3.3–17.2	4.3–19.7
4.5	10	6.0–7.7	14.0–25.8	4.7–6.2	9.0–10.9	6.3–16.6	8.0–9.8	4.1–17.9	5.2–20.6
5.0	11	6.1–7.8	14.9–26.7	4.9–6.2	9.2–11.1	6.9–17.2	8.1–9.9	4.7–18.5	6.0–21.4
5.5	12	6.2–7.8	15.7–27.5	5.0–6.3	9.4–11.2	7.5–17.8	8.3–10.0	5.3–19.1	6.7–22.1
5.9	13	6.3–7.9	16.5–28.3	5.0–6.4	9.5–11.3	8.0–18.3	8.4–10.1	5.8–19.6	7.4–22.8
6.4	14	6.4–8.0	17.2–29.0	5.1–6.4	9.7–11.4	8.5–18.8	8.6–10.2	6.3–20.1	8.0–23.4
6.8	15	6.6–8.1	17.8–29.6	5.2–6.5	9.9–11.5	9.0–19.3	8.7–10.3	6.8–20.6	8.6–24.0
7.3	16	6.7–8.1	18.5–30.2	5.3–6.5	10.0–11.7	9.4–19.7	8.8–10.4	7.2–21.0	9.1–24.5
7.7	17	6.8–8.2	19.0–30.8	5.4–6.6	10.2–11.8	9.8–20.1	9.0–10.4	7.6–21.4	9.7–25.0
8.2	18	6.9–8.3	19.6–31.3	5.5–6.6	10.3–11.9	10.2–20.4	9.1–10.5	8.0–21.8	10.1–25.5
8.6	19	7.0–8.3	20.1–31.8	5.6–6.7	10.5–12.0	10.5–20.8	9.2–10.6	8.4–22.2	10.6–26.0
9.1	20	7.1–8.4	20.6–32.3	5.7–6.7	10.6–12.1	10.9–21.1	9.4–10.7	8.7–22.5	11.0–26.4
9.5	21	7.2–8.5	21.0–32.8	5.7–6.8	10.8–12.2	11.2–21.4	9.5–10.8	9.0–22.8	11.5–26.8
10.0	22	7.3–8.5	21.5–33.2	5.8–6.9	10.9–12.3	11.5–21.7	9.6–10.9	9.3–23.1	11.8–27.2
10.5	23	7.4–8.6	21.9–33.6	5.9–6.9	11.1–12.4	11.8–22.0	9.7–11.0	9.6–23.4	12.2–27.6

10.9	24	7.5–8.7	22.3–34.0	6.0–7.0	11.2–12.5	12.1–22.3	9.8–11.0	9.9–23.7	12.6–27.9
11.4	25	7.6–8.7	22.7–34.4	6.1–7.0	11.3–12.6	12.3–22.6	9.9–11.1	10.2–24.0	12.9–28.3
11.8	26	7.6–8.8	23.0–34.8	6.1–7.1	11.5–12.7	12.6–22.8	10.0–11.2	10.5–24.2	13.3–28.6
12.3	27	7.7–8.8	23.4–35.1	6.2–7.1	11.6–12.9	12.8–23.1	10.1–11.3	10.7–24.5	13.6–28.9
12.7	28	7.8–8.9	23.7–35.5	6.3–7.2	11.7–13.0	13.1–23.3	10.3–11.4	11.0–24.7	13.9–29.2
13.2	29	7.9–9.0	24.1–35.8	6.3–7.2	11.9–13.1	13.3–23.5	10.4–11.5	11.2–25.0	14.2–29.5
13.6	30	8.0–9.0	24.4–36.1	6.4–7.3	12.0–13.2	13.5–23.8	10.5–11.5	11.4–25.2	14.5–29.8
14.1	31	8.1–9.1	24.7–36.4	6.5–7.3	12.1–13.3	13.7–24.0	10.6–11.6	11.6–25.4	14.8–30.1
14.5	32	8.1–9.2	25.0–36.7	6.5–7.4	12.2–13.4	13.9–24.2	10.7–11.7	11.9–25.6	15.0–30.3
15.0	33	8.2–9.2	25.3–37.0	6.6–7.4	12.4–13.5	14.1–24.4	10.8–11.8	12.1–25.8	15.3–30.6
15.5	34	8.3–9.3	25.6–37.3	6.7–7.5	12.5–13.6	14.3–24.6	10.8–11.9	12.3–26.0	15.5–30.8
15.9	35	8.4–9.3	25.9–37.6	6.7–7.5	12.6–13.7	14.5–24.8	10.9–11.9	12.5–26.2	15.8–31.1
16.4	36	8.5–9.4	26.1–37.8	6.8–7.6	12.7–13.8	14.7–24.9	11.0–12.0	12.7–26.4	16.0–31.3
16.8	37	8.5–9.5	26.4–38.1	6.8–7.6	12.8–13.9	14.9–25.1	11.1–12.1	12.8–26.6	16.2–31.6
17.3	38	8.6–9.5	26.6–38.3	6.9–7.7	12.9–13.9	15.1–25.3	11.2–12.2	13.0–26.7	16.5–31.8
17.7	39	8.7–9.6	26.9–38.6	7.0–7.7	13.0–14.0	15.2–25.5	11.3–12.3	13.2–26.9	16.7–32.0
18.2	40	8.7–9.6	27.1–38.8	7.0–7.8	13.1–14.1	15.4–25.6	11.4–12.3	13.4–27.1	16.9–32.2
18.6	41	8.8–9.7	27.4–39.1	7.1–7.8	13.2–14.2	15.6–25.8	11.5–12.4	13.5–27.2	17.1–32.4
19.1	42	8.9–9.8	27.6–39.3	7.1–7.9	13.3–14.3	15.7–25.9	11.6–12.5	13.7–27.4	17.3–32.6
19.5	43	8.9–9.8	27.8–39.5	7.2–7.9	13.4–14.4	15.9–26.1	11.6–12.6	13.8–27.6	17.5–32.8
20.0	44	9.0–9.9	28.0–39.7	7.2–8.0	13.5–14.5	16.0–26.2	11.7–12.6	14.0–27.7	17.7–33.0
20.5	45	9.1–10.0	28.2–39.9	7.3–8.0	13.6–14.6	16.2–26.4	11.8–12.7	14.2–27.9	17.9–33.2
20.9	46	9.1–10.0	28.4–40.1	7.3–8.1	13.7–14.7	16.3–26.5	11.9–12.8	14.3–28.0	18.1–33.4
21.4	47	9.2–10.1	28.6–40.3	7.4–8.1	13.8–14.8	16.5–26.7	11.9–12.9	14.4–28.2	18.3–33.6
21.8	48	9.2–10.1	28.8–40.5	7.4–8.2	13.9–14.9	16.6–26.8	12.0–13.0	14.6–28.3	18.5–33.7
22.3	49	9.3–10.2	29.0–40.7	7.5–8.2	14.0–15.0	16.7–26.9	12.1–13.1	14.7–28.4	18.6–33.9
22.7	50	9.4–10.3	29.2–40.9	7.5–8.3	14.1–15.1	16.9–27.1	12.2–13.1	14.9–28.6	18.8–34.1

(continued)

Table 6.4 (*Continued*)

| | | | | | | CANINE M-MODE REFERENCE RANGES[18] | | | | |
| | | | | | | 95% prediction intervals (mm) | | | | |
kg	Lbs	VS d	LV d	LVWd	VSs	LVs	LVWs	AO	LA
23.2	51	9.4–10.3	29.4–41.1	7.6–8.4	14.2–15.2	17.0–27.2	12.2–13.2	15.0–28.7	19.0–34.2
23.6	52	9.5–10.4	29.6–41.3	7.6–8.4	14.3–15.3	17.1–27.3	12.3–13.3	15.1–28.8	19.1–34.4
24.1	53	9.5–10.5	29.8–41.5	7.7–8.5	14.4–15.4	17.3–27.5	12.4–13.4	15.2–29.0	19.3–34.6
24.5	54	9.6–10.5	30.0–41.6	7.7–8.5	14.5–15.5	17.4–27.6	12.4–13.5	15.4–29.1	19.4–34.7
25.0	55	9.6–10.6	30.1–41.8	7.8–8.6	14.6–15.6	17.5–27.7	12.5–13.5	15.5–29.2	19.6–34.9
25.5	56	9.7–10.7	30.3–42.0	7.8–8.6	14.6–15.7	17.6–27.8	12.6–13.6	15.6–29.3	19.8–35.0
25.9	57	9.7–10.7	30.5–42.1	7.8–8.7	14.7–15.8	17.7–27.9	12.6–13.7	15.7–29.4	19.9–35.2
26.4	58	9.8–10.8	30.6–42.3	7.9–8.7	14.8–15.9	17.8–28.0	12.7–13.8	15.8–29.6	20.1–35.3
26.8	59	9.8–10.9	30.8–42.5	7.9–8.8	14.9–16.0	18.0–28.1	12.8–13.9	16.0–29.7	20.2–35.5
27.3	60	9.9–10.9	30.9–42.6	8.0–8.8	15.0–16.1	18.1–28.3	12.8–13.9	16.1–29.8	20.3–35.6
27.7	61	9.9–11.0	31.1–42.8	8.0–8.9	15.0–16.2	18.2–28.4	12.9–14.0	16.2–29.9	20.5–35.7
28.2	62	10.0–11.0	31.3–42.9	8.0–8.9	15.1–16.3	18.3–28.5	13.0–14.1	16.3–30.0	20.6–35.9
28.6	63	10.0–11.1	31.4–43.1	8.1–9.0	15.2–16.4	18.4–28.6	13.0–14.2	16.4–30.1	20.7–36.0
29.1	64	10.1–11.2	31.6–43.2	8.1–9.1	15.3–16.5	18.5–28.7	13.1–14.3	16.5–30.2	20.9–36.2
29.5	65	10.1–11.2	31.7–43.4	8.2–9.1	15.4–16.6	18.6–28.8	13.1–14.3	16.6–30.3	21.0–36.3
30.0	66	10.2–11.3	31.8–43.5	8.2–9.2	15.4–16.7	18.7–28.9	13.2–14.4	16.7–30.4	21.1–36.4
30.5	67	10.2–11.4	32.0–43.7	8.2–9.2	15.5–16.8	18.8–29.0	13.3–14.5	16.8–30.5	21.3–36.5
30.9	68	10.3–11.4	32.1–43.8	8.3–9.3	15.6–16.9	18.9–29.1	13.3–14.6	16.9–30.6	21.4–36.7
31.4	69	10.3–11.5	32.3–43.9	8.3–9.3	15.7–17.0	19.0–29.2	13.4–14.7	17.0–30.7	21.5–36.8
31.8	70	10.4–11.6	32.4–44.1	8.3–9.4	15.7–17.1	19.1–29.3	13.4–14.7	17.1–30.8	21.6–36.9
32.3	71	10.4–11.6	32.5–44.2	8.4–9.4	15.8–17.2	19.2–29.4	13.5–14.8	17.2–30.9	21.7–37.0
32.7	72	10.4–11.7	32.7–44.4	8.4–9.5	15.9–17.3	19.3–29.5	13.6–14.9	17.3–31.0	21.9–37.1
33.2	73	10.5–11.8	32.8–44.5	8.4–9.5	15.9–17.4	19.3–29.5	13.6–15.0	17.4–31.1	22.0–37.3

33.6	74	10.5–11.8	32.9–44.6	8.5–9.6	16.0–17.5	19.4–29.6	13.7–15.1	17.5–31.2	22.1–37.4
34.1	75	10.6–11.9	33.0–44.7	8.5–9.6	16.1–17.6	19.5–29.7	13.7–15.1	17.6–31.3	22.2–37.5
34.5	76	10.6–12.0	33.2–44.9	8.5–9.7	16.2–17.7	19.6–29.8	13.8–15.2	17.6–31.4	22.3–37.6
35.0	77	10.6–12.0	33.3–45.0	8.6–9.7	16.2–17.7	19.7–29.9	13.8–15.3	17.7–31.4	22.4–37.7
35.5	78	10.7–12.1	33.4–45.1	8.6–9.8	16.3–17.8	19.8–30.0	13.9–15.4	17.8–31.5	22.5–37.8
35.9	79	10.7–12.1	33.5–45.2	8.6–9.8	16.4–17.9	19.9–30.1	13.9–15.4	17.9–31.6	22.6–37.9
36.4	80	10.8–12.2	33.6–45.3	8.7–9.9	16.4–18.0	19.9–30.1	14.0–15.5	18.0–31.7	22.7–38.0
36.8	81	10.8–12.3	33.8–45.5	8.7–10.0	16.5–18.1	20.0–30.2	14.0–15.6	18.1–31.8	22.8–38.1
37.3	82	10.9–12.3	33.9–45.6	8.7–10.0	16.6–18.2	20.1–30.3	14.1–15.7	18.1–31.9	23.0–38.3
37.7	83	10.9–12.4	34.0–45.7	8.8–10.1	16.6–18.3	20.2–30.4	14.2–15.8	18.2–32.0	23.1–38.4
38.2	84	10.9–12.5	34.1–45.8	8.8–10.1	16.7–18.4	20.2–30.5	14.2–15.8	18.3–32.0	23.2–38.5
38.6	85	11.0–12.5	34.2–45.9	8.8–10.2	16.8–18.5	20.3–30.5	14.3–15.9	18.4–32.1	23.2–38.6
39.1	86	11.0–12.6	34.3–46.0	8.9–10.2	16.8–18.6	20.4–30.6	14.3–16.0	18.5–32.2	23.3–38.7
39.5	87	11.0–12.6	34.4–46.1	8.9–10.3	16.9–18.7	20.5–30.7	14.4–16.1	18.5–32.3	23.4–38.8
40.0	88	11.1–12.7	34.5–46.3	8.9–10.3	17.0–18.8	20.5–30.8	14.4–16.1	18.6–32.4	23.5–38.9
40.5	89	11.1–12.8	34.6–46.4	9.0–10.4	17.0–18.9	20.6–30.8	14.5–16.2	18.7–32.4	23.6–39.0
40.9	90	11.2–12.8	34.7–46.5	9.0–10.4	17.1–19.0	20.7–30.9	14.5–16.3	18.8–32.5	23.7–39.0
41.4	91	11.2–12.9	34.8–46.6	9.0–10.5	17.2–19.0	20.8–31.0	14.6–16.4	18.8–32.6	23.8–39.1
41.8	92	11.2–13.0	34.9–46.7	9.1–10.5	17.2–19.1	20.8–31.1	14.6–16.4	18.9–32.7	23.9–39.2
42.3	93	11.3–13.0	35.0–46.8	9.1–10.6	17.3–19.2	20.9–31.1	14.7–16.5	19.0–32.7	24.0–39.3
42.7	94	11.3–13.1	35.1–46.9	9.1–10.6	17.4–19.3	21.0–31.2	14.7–16.6	19.0–32.8	24.1–39.4
43.2	95	11.3–13.1	35.2–47.0	9.2–10.7	17.4–19.4	21.0–31.3	14.8–16.7	19.1–32.9	24.2–39.5
43.6	96	11.4–13.2	35.3–47.1	9.2–10.7	17.5–19.5	21.1–31.4	14.8–16.7	19.2–32.9	24.3–39.6
44.1	97	11.4–13.3	35.4–47.2	9.2–10.8	17.5–19.6	21.2–31.4	14.9–16.8	19.2–33.0	24.3–39.7
44.5	98	11.5–13.3	35.5–47.3	9.2–10.8	17.6–19.7	21.2–31.5	14.9–16.9	19.3–33.1	24.4–39.8
45.0	99	11.5–13.4	35.6–47.4	9.3–10.9	17.7–19.8	21.3–31.6	15.0–16.9	19.4–33.2	24.5–39.9
45.5	100	11.5–13.4	35.7–47.5	9.3–10.9	17.7–19.8	21.4–31.6	15.0–17.0	19.4–33.2	24.6–40.0

(continued)

Table 6.4 (*Continued*)

CANINE M-MODE REFERENCE RANGES[18]

95% prediction intervals (mm)

kg	Lbs	VS d	LV d	LVWd	VSs	LVs	LVWs	AO	LA
45.9	101	11.6–13.5	35.8–47.6	9.3–11.0	17.8–19.9	21.4–31.7	15.1–17.1	19.5–33.3	24.7–40.0
46.4	102	11.6–13.6	35.9–47.7	9.4–11.0	17.8–20.0	21.5–31.8	15.1–17.2	19.6–33.4	24.8–40.1
46.8	103	11.6–13.6	36.0–47.8	9.4–11.1	17.9–20.1	21.6–31.8	15.2–17.2	19.6–33.4	24.8–40.2
47.3	104	11.7–13.7	36.1–47.9	9.4–11.1	18.0–20.2	21.6–31.9	15.2–17.3	19.7–33.5	24.9–40.3
47.7	105	11.7–13.7	36.2–47.9	9.5–11.2	18.0–20.3	21.7–32.0	15.2–17.4	19.8–33.6	25.0–40.4
48.2	106	11.7–13.8	36.3–48.0	9.5–11.2	18.1–20.4	21.7–32.0	15.3–17.5	19.8–33.6	25.1–40.5
48.6	107	11.8–13.9	36.3–48.1	9.5–11.3	18.2–20.5	21.8–32.1	15.3–17.5	19.9–33.7	25.1–40.5
49.1	108	11.8–13.9	36.4–48.2	9.5–11.3	18.2–20.5	21.9–32.1	15.4–17.6	19.9–33.8	25.2–40.6
49.5	109	11.9–14.0	36.5–48.3	9.6–11.4	18.3–20.6	21.9–32.2	15.4–17.7	20.0–33.8	25.3–40.7
50.0	110	11.9–14.0	36.6–48.4	9.6–11.4	18.3–20.7	22.0–32.3	15.5–17.7	20.1–33.9	25.4–40.8
50.5	111	11.9–14.1	36.7–48.5	9.6–11.5	18.4–20.8	22.0–32.3	15.5–17.8	20.1–34.0	25.4–40.9
50.9	112	12.0–14.1	36.8–48.6	9.7–11.5	18.5–20.9	22.1–32.4	15.6–17.9	20.2–34.0	25.5–40.9
51.4	113	12.0–14.2	36.8–48.7	9.7–11.5	18.5–21.0	22.1–32.4	15.6–18.0	20.2–34.1	25.6–41.0
51.8	114	12.0–14.3	36.9–48.7	9.7–11.6	18.6–21.1	22.2–32.5	15.7–18.0	20.3–34.1	25.7–41.1
52.3	115	12.1–14.3	37.0–48.8	9.7–11.6	18.6–21.1	22.2–32.6	15.7–18.1	20.3–34.2	25.7–41.2
52.7	116	12.1–14.4	37.1–48.9	9.8–11.7	18.7–21.2	22.3–32.6	15.8–18.2	20.4–34.3	25.8–41.3
53.2	117	12.1–14.4	37.2–49.0	9.8–11.7	18.7–21.3	22.4–32.7	15.8–18.2	20.4–34.3	25.9–41.3
53.6	118	12.2–14.5	37.2–49.1	9.8–11.8	18.8–21.4	22.4–32.7	15.8–18.3	20.5–34.4	25.9–41.4
54.1	119	12.2–14.5	37.3–49.2	9.8–11.8	18.9–21.5	22.5–32.8	15.9–18.4	20.6–34.4	26.0–41.5
54.5	120	12.2–14.6	37.4–49.2	9.9–11.9	18.9–21.6	22.5–32.9	15.9–18.4	20.6–34.5	26.1–41.6

55.0	121	12.3–14.7	37.5–49.3	9.9–11.9	19.0–21.6	22.6–32.9	16.0–18.5	20.7–34.6	26.1–41.6
55.5	122	12.3–14.7	37.5–49.4	9.9–12.0	19.0–21.7	22.6–33.0	16.0–18.6	20.7–34.6	26.2–41.7
55.9	123	12.3–14.8	37.6–49.5	10.0–12.0	19.1–21.8	22.7–33.0	16.1–18.7	20.8–34.7	26.3–41.8
56.4	124	12.4–14.8	37.7–49.6	10.0–12.1	19.1–21.9	22.7–33.1	16.1–18.7	20.8–34.7	26.3–41.8
56.8	125	12.4–14.9	37.8–49.6	10.0–12.1	19.2–22.0	22.8–33.1	16.2–18.8	20.9–34.8	26.4–41.9
57.3	126	12.4–14.9	37.8–49.7	10.0–12.2	19.3–22.1	22.8–33.2	16.2–18.9	20.9–34.8	26.5–42.0
57.7	127	12.5–15.0	37.9–49.8	10.1–12.2	19.3–22.1	22.9–33.2	16.2–18.9	21.0–34.9	26.5–42.1
58.2	128	12.5–15.1	38.0–49.9	10.1–12.3	19.4–22.2	22.9–33.3	16.3–19.0	21.0–35.0	26.6–42.1
58.6	129	12.5–15.1	38.0–49.9	10.1–12.3	19.4–22.3	23.0–33.3	16.3–19.1	21.1–35.0	26.6–42.2
59.1	130	12.6–15.2	38.1–50.0	10.1–12.3	19.5–22.4	23.0–33.4	16.4–19.1	21.1–35.1	26.7–42.3
59.5	131	12.6–15.2	38.2–50.1	10.2–12.4	19.5–22.5	23.1–33.5	16.4–19.2	21.2–35.1	26.8–42.3
60.0	132	12.6–15.3	38.3–50.2	10.2–12.4	19.6–22.6	23.1–33.5	16.5–19.3	21.2–35.2	26.8–42.4
60.5	133	12.7–15.3	38.3–50.2	10.2–12.5	19.7–22.6	23.2–33.6	16.5–19.3	21.2–35.2	26.9–42.5
60.9	134	12.7–15.4	38.4–50.3	10.3–12.5	19.7–22.7	23.2–33.6	16.6–19.4	21.3–35.3	26.9–42.5
61.4	135	12.7–15.4	38.5–50.4	10.3–12.6	19.8–22.8	23.2–33.7	16.6–19.5	21.3–35.3	27.0–42.6
61.8	136	12.7–15.5	38.5–50.5	10.3–12.6	19.8–22.9	23.3–33.7	16.6–19.5	21.4–35.4	27.1–42.7
62.3	137	12.8–15.6	38.6–50.5	10.3–12.7	19.9–23.0	23.3–33.8	16.7–19.6	21.4–35.4	27.1–42.7
62.7	138	12.8–15.6	38.7–50.6	10.4–12.7	19.9–23.0	23.4–33.8	16.7–19.7	21.5–35.5	27.2–42.8
63.2	139	12.8–15.7	38.7–50.7	10.4–12.8	20.0–23.1	23.4–33.9	16.8–19.7	21.5–35.5	27.2–42.9
63.6	140	12.9–15.7	38.8–50.8	10.4–12.8	20.0–23.2	23.5–33.9	16.8–19.8	21.6–35.6	27.3–42.9
64.1	141	12.9–15.8	38.8–50.8	10.4–12.8	20.1–23.3	23.5–34.0	16.8–19.9	21.6–35.7	27.3–43.0
64.5	142	12.9–15.8	38.9–50.9	10.5–12.9	20.1–23.4	23.6–34.0	16.9–19.9	21.6–35.7	27.4–43.1
65.0	143	13.0–15.9	39.0–51.0	10.5–12.9	20.2–23.4	23.6–34.1	16.9–20.0	21.7–35.8	27.4–43.1
65.5	144	13.0–15.9	39.0–51.0	10.5–13.0	20.3–23.5	23.6–34.1	17.0–20.1	21.7–35.8	27.5–43.2

(continued)

Table 6.4 (*Continued*)

					CANINE M-MODE REFERENCE RANGES[18]				
					95% prediction intervals (mm)				
kg	Lbs	VS d	LV d	LVWd	VSs	LVs	LVWs	AO	LA
65.9	145	13.0–16.0	39.1–51.1	10.5–13.0	20.3–23.6	23.7–34.2	17.0–20.1	21.8–35.9	27.6–43.2
66.4	146	13.1–16.0	39.2–51.2	10.6–13.1	20.4–23.7	23.7–34.2	17.1–20.2	21.8–35.9	27.6–43.3
66.8	147	13.1–16.1	39.2–51.2	10.6–13.1	20.4–23.8	23.8–34.3	17.1–20.3	21.9–36.0	27.7–43.4
67.3	148	13.1–16.1	39.3–51.3	10.6–13.2	20.5–23.8	23.8–34.3	17.1–20.3	21.9–36.0	27.7–43.4
67.7	149	13.2–16.2	39.3–51.4	10.6–13.2	20.5–23.9	23.8–34.3	17.2–20.4	21.9–36.1	27.8–43.5
68.2	150	13.2–16.3	39.4–51.4	10.7–13.2	20.6–24.0	23.9–34.4	17.2–20.5	22.0–36.1	27.8–43.6
68.6	151	13.2–16.3	39.4–51.5	10.7–13.3	20.6–24.1	23.9–34.4	17.3–20.5	22.0–36.2	27.9–43.6
69.1	152	13.2–16.4	39.5–51.6	10.7–13.3	20.7–24.1	24.0–34.5	17.3–20.6	22.1–36.2	27.9–43.7
69.5	153	13.3–16.4	39.6–51.6	10.7–13.4	20.7–24.2	24.0–34.5	17.3–20.6	22.1–36.3	28.0–43.7
70.0	154	13.3–16.5	39.6–51.7	10.8–13.4	20.8–24.3	24.0–34.6	17.4–20.7	22.1–36.3	28.0–43.8
70.5	155	13.3–16.5	39.7–51.8	10.8–13.5	20.8–24.4	24.1–34.6	17.4–20.8	22.2–36.3	28.1–43.9
70.9	156	13.4–16.6	39.7–51.8	10.8–13.5	20.9–24.5	24.1–34.7	17.5–20.8	22.2–36.4	28.1–43.9
71.4	157	13.4–16.6	39.8–51.9	10.8–13.5	20.9–24.5	24.2–34.7	17.5–20.9	22.2–36.4	28.2–44.0
71.8	158	13.4–16.7	39.8–52.0	10.9–13.6	21.0–24.6	24.2–34.8	17.6–21.0	22.3–36.5	28.2–44.0
72.3	159	13.5–16.7	39.9–52.0	10.9–13.6	21.0–24.7	24.2–34.8	17.6–21.0	22.3–36.5	28.3–44.1
72.7	160	13.5–16.8	40.0–52.1	10.9–13.7	21.1–24.8	24.3–34.9	17.6–21.1	22.4–36.6	28.3–44.2
73.2	161	13.5–16.8	40.0–52.2	10.9–13.7	21.1–24.8	24.3–34.9	17.7–21.2	22.4–36.6	28.3–44.2
73.6	162	13.6–16.9	40.1–52.2	11.0–13.8	21.2–24.9	24.3–34.9	17.7–21.2	22.4–36.7	28.4–44.3
74.1	163	13.6–16.9	40.1–52.3	11.0–13.8	21.3–25.0	24.4–35.0	17.8–21.3	22.5–36.7	28.4–44.3
74.5	164	13.6–17.0	40.2–52.3	11.0–13.8	21.3–25.1	24.4–35.0	17.8–21.3	22.5–36.8	28.5–44.4
75.0	165	13.6–17.0	40.2–52.4	11.0–13.9	21.4–25.1	24.4–35.1	17.8–21.4	22.5–36.8	28.5–44.4

75.5	166	13.7–17.1	40.3–52.5	11.1–13.9	21.4–25.2	24.5–35.1	17.9–21.5	22.6–36.9	28.6–44.5
75.9	167	13.7–17.1	40.3–52.5	11.1–14.0	21.5–25.3	24.5–35.2	17.9–21.5	22.6–36.9	28.6–44.6
76.4	168	13.7–17.2	40.4–52.6	11.1–14.0	21.5–25.4	24.6–35.2	18.0–21.6	22.6–37.0	28.7–44.6
76.8	169	13.8–17.2	40.4–52.6	11.1–14.1	21.6–25.4	24.6–35.2	18.0–21.7	22.7–37.0	28.7–44.7
77.3	170	13.8–17.3	40.5–52.7	11.2–14.1	21.6–25.5	24.6–35.3	18.0–21.7	22.7–37.0	28.8–44.7
77.7	171	13.8–17.3	40.5–52.8	11.2–14.1	21.7–25.6	24.7–35.3	18.1–21.8	22.7–37.1	28.8–44.8
78.2	172	13.8–17.4	40.6–52.8	11.2–14.2	21.7–25.7	24.7–35.4	18.1–21.8	22.8–37.1	28.8–44.8
78.6	173	13.9–17.4	40.6–52.9	11.2–14.2	21.8–25.7	24.7–35.4	18.1–21.9	22.8–37.2	28.9–44.9
79.1	174	13.9–17.5	40.7–52.9	11.3–14.3	21.8–25.8	24.8–35.5	18.2–22.0	22.8–37.2	28.9–45.0
79.5	175	13.9–17.5	40.7–53.0	11.3–14.3	21.9–25.9	24.8–35.5	18.2–22.0	22.9–37.3	29.0–45.0
80.0	176	14.0–17.6	40.8–53.1	11.3–14.4	21.9–26.0	24.8–35.5	18.3–22.1	22.9–37.3	29.0–45.1
80.5	177	14.0–17.6	40.8–53.1	11.3–14.4	22.0–26.0	24.9–35.6	18.3–22.1	22.9–37.4	29.0–45.1
80.9	178	14.0–17.7	40.9–53.2	11.3–14.4	22.0–26.1	24.9–35.6	18.3–22.2	23.0–37.4	29.1–45.2
81.4	179	14.0–17.8	40.9–53.2	11.4–14.5	22.1–26.2	24.9–35.7	18.4–22.3	23.0–37.4	29.1–45.2
81.8	180	14.1–17.8	41.0–53.3	11.4–14.5	22.1–26.3	25.0–35.7	18.4–22.3	23.0–37.5	29.2–45.3
82.3	181	14.1–17.9	41.0–53.4	11.4–14.6	22.2–26.3	25.0–35.7	18.5–22.4	23.1–37.5	29.2–45.3
82.7	182	14.1–17.9	41.1–53.4	11.4–14.6	22.2–26.4	25.0–35.8	18.5–22.5	23.1–37.6	29.2–45.4
83.2	183	14.2–18.0	41.1–53.5	11.5–14.6	22.3–26.5	25.1–35.8	18.5–22.5	23.1–37.6	29.3–45.4
83.6	184	14.2–18.0	41.2–53.5	11.5–14.7	22.3–26.6	25.1–35.9	18.6–22.6	23.2–37.7	29.3–45.5
84.1	185	14.2–18.1	41.2–53.6	11.5–14.7	22.4–26.6	25.1–35.9	18.6–22.6	23.2–37.7	29.4–45.5
84.5	186	14.2–18.1	41.2–53.6	11.5–14.8	22.4–26.7	25.1–35.9	18.7–22.7	23.2–37.7	29.4–45.6
85.0	187	14.3–18.2	41.3–53.7	11.6–14.8	22.5–26.8	25.2–36.0	18.7–22.8	23.2–37.8	29.4–45.6
85.5	188	14.3–18.2	41.3–53.7	11.6–14.8	22.5–26.8	25.2–36.0	18.7–22.8	23.3–37.8	29.5–45.7
85.9	189	14.3–18.2	41.4–53.8	11.6–14.9	22.6–26.9	25.2–36.1	18.8–22.9	23.3–37.9	29.5–45.8
86.4	190	14.4–18.3	41.4–53.9	11.6–14.9	22.6–27.0	25.3–36.1	18.8–22.9	23.3–37.9	29.6–45.8

(continued)

Table 6.4 (*Continued*)

				CANINE M-MODE REFERENCE RANGES[18]						
				95% prediction intervals (mm)						
kg	Lbs	VS d	LV d	LVWd	VSs	LVs	LVWs	AO	LA
86.8	191	14.4–18.3	41.5–53.9	11.6–15.0	22.7–27.1	25.3–36.1	18.8–23.0	23.4–37.9	29.6–45.9
87.3	192	14.4–18.4	41.5–54.0	11.7–15.0	22.7–27.1	25.3–36.2	18.9–23.1	23.4–38.0	29.6–45.9
87.7	193	14.4–18.4	41.6–54.0	11.7–15.1	22.8–27.2	25.3–36.2	18.9–23.1	23.4–38.0	29.7–46.0
88.2	194	14.5–18.5	41.6–54.1	11.7–15.1	22.8–27.3	25.4–36.3	19.0–23.2	23.4–38.1	29.7–46.0
88.6	195	14.5–18.5	41.6–54.1	11.7–15.1	22.8–27.3	25.4–36.3	19.0–23.2	23.5–38.1	29.7–46.1
89.1	196	14.5–18.6	41.7–54.2	11.8–15.2	22.9–27.4	25.4–36.3	19.0–23.3	23.5–38.2	29.8–46.1
89.5	197	14.6–18.6	41.7–54.2	11.8–15.2	22.9–27.5	25.5–36.4	19.1–23.4	23.5–38.2	29.8–46.2
90.0	198	14.6–18.7	41.8–54.3	11.8–15.3	23.0–27.6	25.5–36.4	19.1–23.4	23.5–38.2	29.8–46.2
90.5	199	14.6–18.7	41.8–54.3	11.8–15.3	23.0–27.6	25.5–36.5	19.1–23.5	23.6–38.3	29.9–46.3
90.9	200	14.6–18.8	41.8–54.4	11.9–15.3	23.1–27.7	25.5–36.5	19.2–23.5	23.6–38.3	29.9–46.3

To use this table, look up the weight of the dog in the first column on the left, go across the row to find the 95% prediction interval for the parameter in question. Parameters are listed across the top of the table. This is a generic reference table, and most dogs will fit into these ranges. Breed-specific references are provided in the table.

Example: Dog's weight = 35 kg; dog's LVIDd from the echo = 45.2 mm.

In the row corresponding to body weight 35 kg, the LVIDd has a range of 38.4 mm to 39.9 mm.

Therefore, this dog's LVIDd is increased in size.

Data from:

Goncalves, A.C., Orton, E.C., Boon, J.A., et al. (2002) Linear, logarithmic, and polynomial models of M-mode echocardiographic measurements in dogs. *Am. J. Vet. Res.*, **63**, 994–999.

LV = left ventricle; VS = ventricular septum; LVW = left ventricular wall; d = diastole; s = systole; AO = aorta; LA = left atrium; kg = kilogram; lbs = pounds; mm = millimeter.

Table 6.5 Normalized reference ranges for parameters of size in the dog.

M-mode parameter	Exponent	95% CI
IVSd (cm)	0.241	0.29–0.59
LVIDd (cm)	0.294	1.27–1.85
LVWd (cm)	0.232	0.29–0.60
IVSs (cm)	0.240	0.43–0.79
LVIDs (cm)	0.315	0.71–1.26
LVWs (cm)	0.222	0.48–0.87
LA (cm)	0.345	0.63–0.96
Ao (cm)	0.341	0.59–0.97

Normalized reference ranges means that the 95% CI for a parameter is the same for all sizes of dogs, they have been normalized. To use this table, you must use this equation:

Normalized value = M-mode measurement (cm)/(weight $(kg)^{exponent}$)

Example: LVIDd = 3.4 cm, dog's weight = 23 kg
Normalized value = $3.4/23^{.294}$
Normalized value = 1.39
Normalized reference range for LVIDd = 1.27 – 1.85
Therefore, an LVIDd of 3.4 cm in this 23 kg dog is normal

IVS = interventricular septum; LVID = left ventricular internal diameter; LVW = left ventricular wall; d = diastole; s = systole; LA = left atrium; Ao = aorta; cm = centimeter.
Data from:
Cornell, C., Kittleson, M., and Della Torre, P. (2004) Allometric scaling of M-mode cardiac measurements in normal adult dogs. *J. Vet. Intern. Med.*, **18**, 311–321.

Table 6.6 Echocardiographic reference ranges for parameters unrelated to body size in the dog.

Parameter	95% CI
Left ventricular ejection time (LVET) (ms)	161–195
Pre-ejection period (PEP) (ms)	20–94
PEP/LVET	0.1-0.54
LA/AO	0.83–1.13
EPSS (mm)	0.30–7.7
FS (%)	33–46
IVSd/LVIDd	0.22–0.34
HR	49–146

Parameters of function, ratios and EPSS are independent of body size and weight. Regardless of size, most dogs should fall within these 95% confidence intervals. When breed-specific references are available they should be used instead.
IVSd = interventricular septum in diastole; LVIDd = left ventricular internal dimension in diastole; FS = fractional shortening; LA = left atrium; AO = aorta; HR = heart rate.
Data from:
Boon, J., Wingfield, W., and Miller, C. (1983) Echocardiographic indices in the normal *dog. Vet. Rad.*, **24**, 214–221.
Boon, J. (2013) *Veterinary Echocardiography*, Wiley Blackwell, Philadelphia.

References: Breed-Specific Echocardiographic Reference Ranges

The following includes most breed-specific reference ranges currently available.

Atkins, C. and Snyder, P. (1992) Systolic time intervals and their derivatives for evaluation of cardiac function. *J. Vet. Intern. Med.*, **2**, 55–63.

Baade, H., Schober, K., and Oechtering, G. (2002) Echocardiographic reference values in West Highland white terriers with special regard to right heart function. *Tierarztl. Prax.*, **30**, 172–179.

Bavegems, V., Duchateau, L., Sys, S.U., *et al.* (2007) Echocardiographic reference values in whippets. *Vet. Radiol. Ultrasound*, **48**, 230–238.

Bayón, A., Fernández del Palacio, J., Montes, A., *et al.* (1994) M-mode echocardiography study in growing Spanish mastiffs. *J. Small Anim. Pract.*, **35**, 473–479.

Boon, J., Wingfield, W., and Miller, C. (1983) Echocardiographic indices in the normal dog. *Vet. Radiol. Ultrasound*, **24**, 214–221.

Brown, D.J., Rush, J.E., MacGregor, J., *et al.* (2003) M-mode echocardiographic ratio indices in normal dogs, cats, and horses: A novel quantitative method. *J. Vet. Intern. Med.*, **17**, 653–662.

Calvert, C.A. and Brown, J. (1986) Use of M-mode echocardiography in the diagnosis of congestive cardiomyopathy in Doberman Pinschers. *J. Am. Vet. Med. Assoc.*, **189**, 293–297.

Cornell, C.C., Kittleson, M.D., and Della Torre, P.D. (2004) Allometric scaling of M-mode cardiac measurements in normal adult dogs. *J. Vet. Intern. Med.*, **18**, 311–321.

Crippa, L., Ferro, E., Melloni, E., *et al.* (1992) Echocardiographic parameters and indices in the normal Beagle dog. *Lab. Anim.*, **26**, 190–195.

Cunningham, S.M., Rush, J.E., Freeman, L., *et al.* (2008) Echocardiographic ratio indices in overtly healthy Boxer dogs screened for heart disease. *J. Vet. Intern. Med.*, **22**, 924–930.

Della Toree, P.K., Kirby, A.C., Church, D.B., *et al.* (2000) Echocardiographic measurements in greyhounds, whippets, and Italian greyhounds – dogs with similar conformation but different size. *Aust. Vet. J.*, **78**, 49–55.

de Madron, E. (1983) M-mode echocardiography in the dog. *Ecole Nationale Veterinaire d'Alfort*, 76.

Goncalves, A.C., Orton, E.C., Boon, J.A., *et al.* (2002) Linear, logarithmic, and polynomial models of M-mode echocardiographic measurements in dogs. *Am. J. Vet. Res.*, **63**, 994–999.

Gooding, J., Robinson, W., and Mews, G. (1986) Echocardiographic assessment of left ventricular dimensions in clinically normal English Cocker Spaniels. *Am. J. Vet. Res.*, **47**, 296–300.

Hall, D.J., Cornell, C.C., Crawford, S., *et al.* (2008) Meta-analysis of normal canine echocardiographic dimensional data using ratio indices. *J. Vet. Cardiol.*, **10**, 11–23.

Herrtage, M.E. (1994) Echocardiographic measurements in the normal Boxer. European Society of Veterinary Internal Medicine Congress, 172.

Jacobson, J.H., Boon, J.A., and Bright, J.M. (2013) An echocardiographic study of healthy Border Collies with normal references ranges for the breed. *J. Vet. Cardiol.*, **15**, 123–130.

Kayar, A., Gonul, R., Or, M., *et al.* (2006) M-mode echocardiographic parameters and indices in the normal German Shepherd dog. *Vet. Radiol. Ultrasound*, **47**, 482–486.

Kayar, A., Ozkan, C., Iskefli, O., *et al.* (2014) Measurement of M-mode echocardiographic parameters in healthy adult Van cats. *Jap. J. Vet. Res.*, **62**, 5–15.

Koch, J., Pedersen, H.D., Jensen, A.L., *et al.* (1996) M-mode echocardiographic diagnosis of dilated cardiomyopathy in giant breed dogs. *J. Vet. Med. Assoc.*, **43**, 297–304.

Lobo, L., Canada, N., Bussadori, C., *et al.* (2008) Transthoracic echocardiography in Estrela Mountain dogs: Reference values for the breed. *Vet. J.*, **177**, 250–259.

Morrison, S.A., Moise, N., Scarlett, J., *et al.* (1992) Effect of breed and body weight on echocardiographic values in four breeds of dogs of differing somatotype. *J. Vet. Intern. Med.*, **6**, 220–224.

Lonsdale, R.A., Labuc, R., and Robertson, I.D. (1998) Echocardiographic parameters in training compared with non-training greyhounds. *Vet. Radiol. Ultrasound*, **39**, 325–330.

Mashiro, I., Nelson, R.R., Cohn, J.N., *et al.* (1976) Ventricular dimensions measured noninvasively by echocardiography in the awake dog. *J. Appl. Physiol.*, **41**, 953–959.

Muzzi, R.A.L., Muzzi, L.A.L., Baracat de Araujo, R., *et al.* (2006) Echocardiographic indices in normal German Shepherd dogs. *J. Vet. Sci.*, **7**, 193–198.

Page, A., Edmunds, G., and Atwell, R.B. (1993) Echocardiographic values in the greyhound. *Aust. Vet. J.*, **70**, 361–364.

Pipers, F.S., Andrysco, R.M., and Hamlin, R.L. (1978) A totally noninvasive method for obtaining systolic time intervals in the dog. *Am. J. Vet. Res.*, **39**, 1822–1826.

Simpson, K.E., Devine, B.C., Woolley, R., *et al.* (2008) Timing of left heart base descent in dogs with dilated cardiomyopathy and normal dogs. *Vet. Radiol. Ultrasound*, **49**, 287–294.

Sisson, D. and Schaeffer, D. (1991) Changes in linear dimensions of the heart, relative to body weight, as measured by M-mode echocardiography in growing dogs. *Am. J. Vet. Res.*, **52**, 1591–1596.

Sleeper, M.M., Henthorn, P.S., Vijayasarathy, C., *et al.* Dilated cardiomyopathy in juvenile Portuguese water dogs. *J. Vet. Intern. Med.*, **16**, 52–62.

Snyder, P.S., Sato, T., and Atkins, C.E. (1995) A comparison of echocardiographic indices of the nonracing, healthy greyhound to reference values from other breeds. *Vet. Radiol. Ultrasound*, **36**, 387–392.

Une, S., Terashita, A., Nakaichi, M., *et al.* (2004) Morphological and functional standard parameters of echocardiogram in beagles. *J. Jpn. Vet. Med. Assoc.*, **57**, 793–798.

Vollmar, A.C. (1999) Use of echocardiography in the diagnosis of dilated cardiomyopathy in Irish wolfhounds. *J. Am. Anim. Hosp. Assoc.*, **35**, 279–283.

Vollmar, A.C. (1999) Echocardiographic measurements in the Irish wolfhound: reference values for the breed. *J. Am. Anim. Hosp. Assoc.*, **35**, 271–277.

Vollmar, A. (1998) Echocardiographic examinations in Deerhounds, reference values for deerhounds. *Kleintierpraxis*, **43**, 497–508.

Voros, K., Hetyey, C., Reiczigel, J., *et al.* (2009) M-mode and two-dimensional echocardiographic reference values for three Hungarian dog breeds: Hungarian Vizsla, Mudi and Hungarian Greyhound. *Acta Vet. Hungar.*, **57** (2), 217–227.

Yamato, R.J., Larsson, M., Mirandola, R.M.S., *et al.* (2006) Echocardiographic parameters in unidimensional mode from clinically normal miniature poodle dogs. *Ciencia Rural*, **36**, 142–148.

Chapter 7 Echocardiographic Features of Common Acquired Heart Diseases

Degenerative Mitral Valve Disease

- Features
  - Mitral valve irregularities (see Figures and Videos 7.1–7.5)
    - May not be appreciated in early stages
    - Possible leaflet prolapse
      - Leaflet(s) bend back into the left atrium
      - May be due to stretching of chordae or rupture of minor chordae
      - Leaflet tip pointing straight back into the left atrium during systole, or doubling back on itself into the left ventricular outflow tract during diastole, is consistent with rupture of a major chordae
  - Left ventricular dilation
    - Degree of dilation correlates to the degree of regurgitation (see Figures and Videos 7.1–7.5)

Two-Dimensional and M-Mode Echocardiography for the Small Animal Practitioner, Second Edition. June A. Boon.
© 2017 John Wiley & Sons, Inc. Published 2017 by John Wiley & Sons, Inc.
Companion Website: www.wiley.com/go/boon/two-dimensional

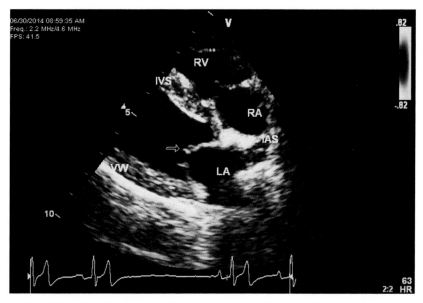

Figure 7.1 Chronic valve disease. This right parasternal four-chamber view shows no obvious dilation of the left ventricle or atrium. The mitral valve has a small club-like increase in thickness at the tip of the anterior leaflet (arrow) and to a lesser extent the posterior leaflet. Left ventricular function appears normal on the video with at least a 30% change in diameter. These minimal changes are consistent with mild degenerative valve disease and minimal to mild mitral regurgitation. For details of abbreviations used in the figures, see the Glossary.

Video 7.1

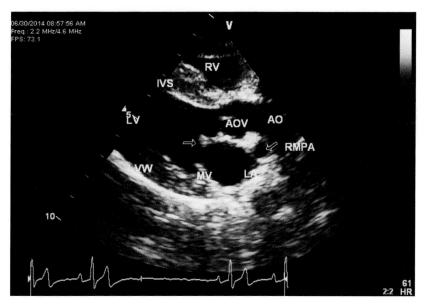

Figure 7.2 Chronic valve disease. This right parasternal inflow outflow view shows no obvious dilation of the left ventricle or atrium. The mitral valve has a small club-like increase in thickness at the tip of the anterior leaflet (arrow). Left ventricular function appears normal on the video with at least a 30% change in diameter. These minimal changes are consistent with mild degenerative valve disease and minimal to mild mitral regurgitation.

Video 7.2

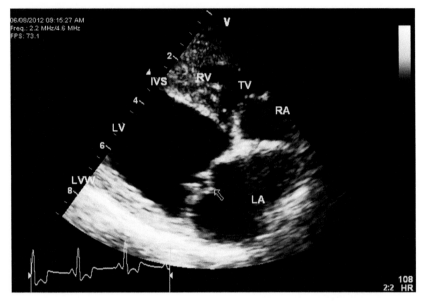

Figure 7.3 Chronic valve disease. This right parasternal four-chamber view of the heart shows mild to moderate left ventricular and left atrial dilation and mild mitral valve prolapse (arrow). Left ventricular function subjectively appears adequate on the video.

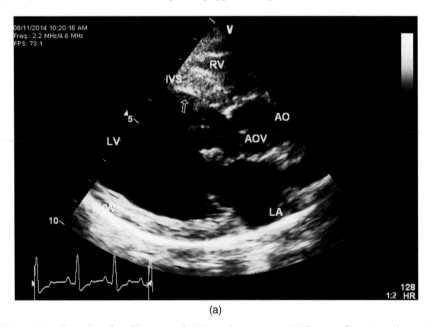

(a)

Figure 7.4 Chronic valve disease. (a,b) This right parasternal inflow outflow view shows at least moderate left ventricular and left atrial dilation. (a) A thickened mitral valve (which should be evaluated during diastole); (b) The septal leaflet prolapsing significantly (arrow) (evaluated during systole). Left ventricular systolic function appears adequate with hyperdynamic motion in the video.

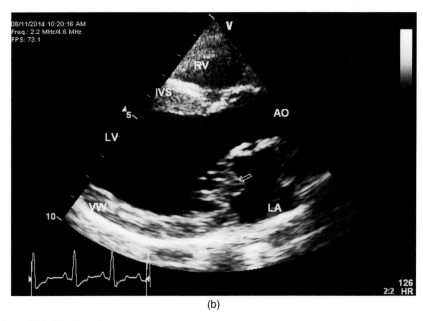

(b)

Figure 7.4 (*Continued*)

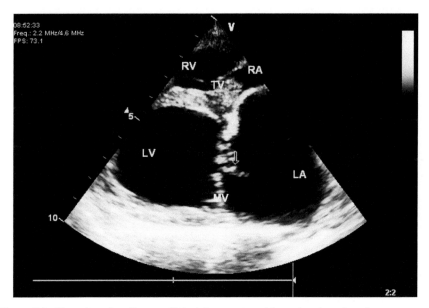

Figure 7.5 Chronic valve disease. This right parasternal four-chamber view shows significant left ventricular and left atrial dilation. The mitral valve is thickened and the septal leaflet points back into the left atrial chamber (arrow), consistent with rupture of a major chordae tendineae.

Video 7.5

- ■ Early stages may show no dilation (remodeling) (see Figure and Video 7.1)
- ○ Left atrial dilation
  - ■ Degree of dilation correlates to the degree of regurgitation (see Figures and Videos 7.1–7.7)
  - ■ Early stages may show no dilation (remodeling) (see Figure and Video 7.1)
- ○ Normal EPSS
- ○ Function may be normal, elevated or depressed
  - ■ If contractility is normal the increased preload results in a normal systolic chamber size and elevated fractional shortening
  - ■ If contractility is depressed then the systolic chamber size is increased and fractional shortening is normal or low
    - ▫ Always rule out high blood pressure as a cause of a large systolic left ventricular chamber size and poor function

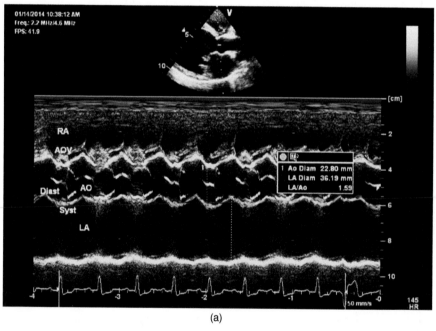

(a)

Figure 7.6 Chronic valve disease. (a) The aorta left atrium M-mode shows a dilated left atrial chamber. The LA:AO is 1.59. Arrows indicate the aortic valve in diastole (left arrow) and systole (right arrow), while the dotted line and calipers show where measurements were made; (b, and Video 7.6) This transverse image of the aorta and left atrium shows a large left atrial chamber. The LA:AO ratio is 3.35. The presence of a pulmonary vein makes estimating the location of the left atrial wall somewhat subjective. In this image it may be a bit further down, but the atrial size is at least 31 mm.

Video 7.6

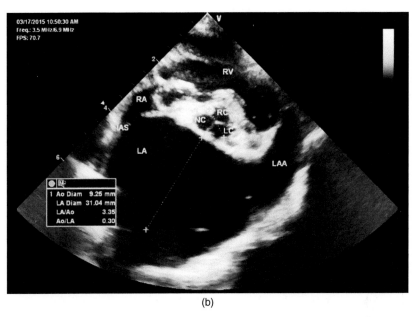

(b)

Figure 7.6 (*Continued*)

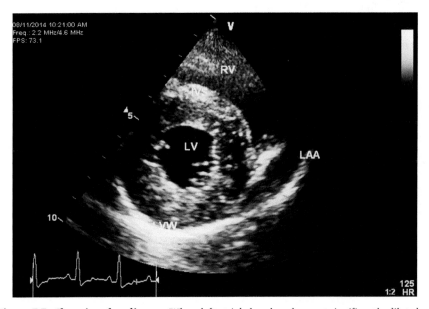

Figure 7.7 Chronic valve disease. When left atrial chambers become significantly dilated the left auricle can be seen to the right side of the transverse left ventricular chamber. Do not confuse this fluid-filled space with pericardial effusion, which would extend to below the left ventricular wall.

Video 7.7

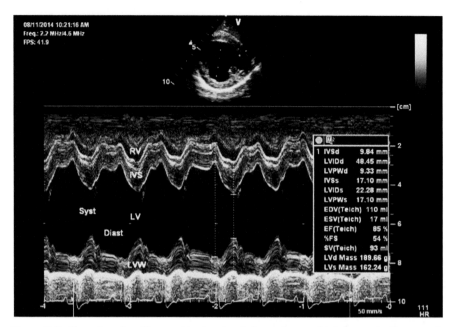

Figure 7.8 Chronic valve disease. The fractional shortening on this left ventricular M-mode is elevated (54%), and the systolic dimension (LVIDs) is normal for a dog of this size. These findings are consistent and expected in a heart with preserved left ventricular contractility. The green calipers and dotted lines show where measurements were made.

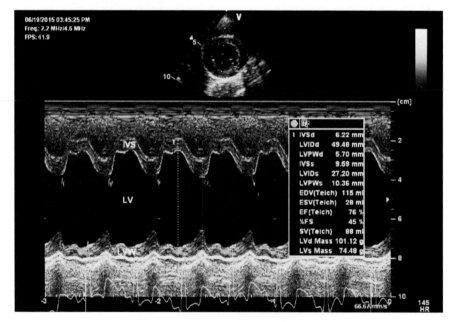

Figure 7.9 Chronic valve disease. Left ventricular function is depressed in the M-mode. Despite normal fractional shortening of 45% the systolic dimension is not normal for a dog of this size. This depressed function may be due to poor contractility or elevated afterload, or a combination of the two.

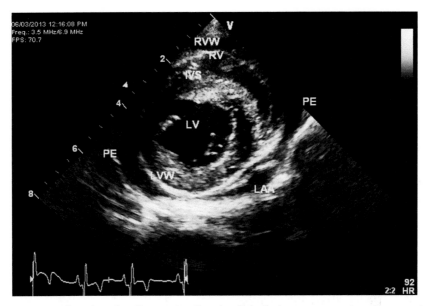

Figure 7.10 Chronic valve disease. Small pericardial effusions may sometimes be seen with advanced degenerative valve disease. On this transverse view of the left ventricular chamber, the black fluid space is seen around the chambers. The small oval-shaped structure to the right side of the left ventricle is the enlarged left atrial appendage (also see Figure and Video 7.7).

Video 7.10

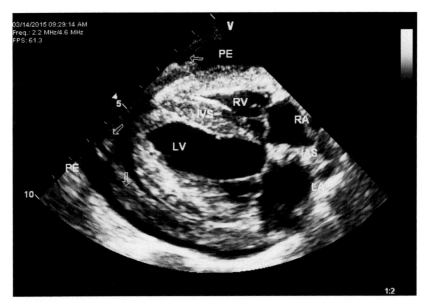

Figure 7.11 Chronic valve disease. Occasionally, left atrial rupture can occur secondary to the chronic left atrial dilation. On this right parasternal four-chamber view a fibrinous layer of thrombus is seen in the pericardial sac (green arrows).

Video 7.11

- ○ Other findings may include:
  - ■ Mild pericardial effusion (see Figure and Video 7.10)
    - □ Fluid seen between the left ventricular wall and pericardial sac
    - □ Usually trace to mild amounts
  - ■ Ruptured left atrium (see Figure and Video 7.11)
    - □ Thrombus in the pericardial sac forms fibrinous layers

Hypertrophic Cardiomyopathy

- • Features
  - ○ Concentric left ventricular hypertrophy (see Figures and Videos 7.12–7.16)
    - ■ This may be symmetric or asymmetric
  - ○ The septum usually extends down into the left ventricular outflow tract, often forming part of the obstruction to outflow (see Figure and Video 7.13)
  - ○ Left atrium may be normal or dilated (see Figures and Videos 7.12–7.14)
    - ■ A large left atrium with left ventricular hypertrophy implies diastolic dysfunction (delayed relaxation)
  - ○ Systolic anterior mitral valve motion (SAM) with obstruction to outflow (see Figures and Videos 7.14, 7.17)
  - ○ Function usually elevated until end-stage

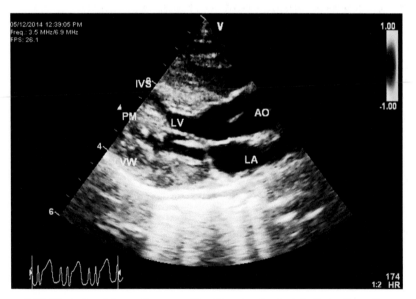

Video 7.12

Figure 7.12 Hypertrophic cardiomyopathy. Hypertrophy that similarly affects the interventricular septum and left ventricular wall is described as symmetric. On this long-axis inflow outflow view there is symmetric hypertrophy of the wall and septum, as well as a prominent and possibly hypertrophied papillary muscle.

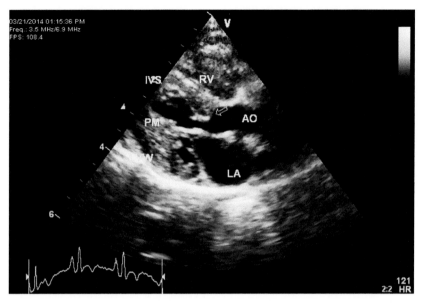

Figure 7.13 Hypertrophic cardiomyopathy. Hypertrophy involving primarily the base of the interventricular septum (arrow) is shown here. The ventricular side of the septum in the outflow tract (arrow) is bright, and is thought to be secondary to the systolic anterior motion seen often in hypertrophic obstructive cardiomyopathy (the "kissing lesion"). Left atrial size is normal in this cat.

Video 7.13

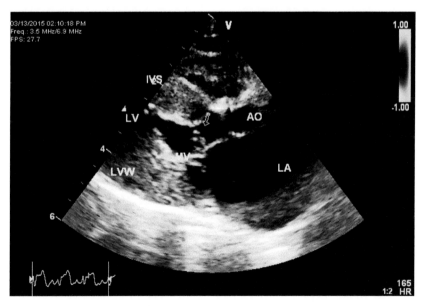

Figure 7.14 Hypertrophic cardiomyopathy. Hypertrophy may be asymmetric. In this case, the left ventricular wall and associated papillary muscle are thicker than the septum. Scan to a transverse view to verify the asymmetry as poor technique may create this appearance too. The left atrium is dilated. The arrow is pointing at systolic anterior mitral valve motion.

Video 7.14

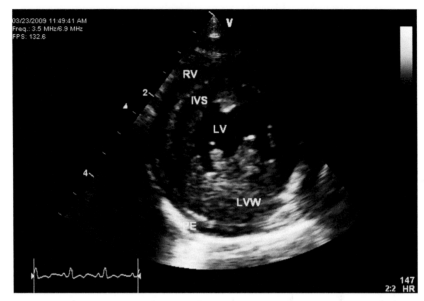

Figure 7.15 **Hypertrophic cardiomyopathy.** Asymmetric hypertrophy is seen on this transverse view of the left ventricle. The left ventricular wall is much thicker than the septum, and the papillary muscles are prominent.

Video 7.15

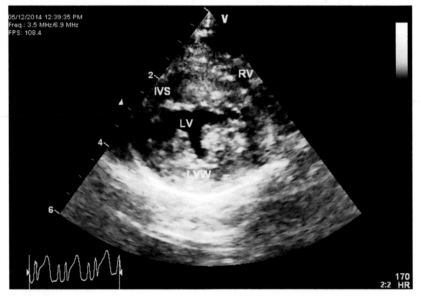

Figure 7.16 **Hypertrophic cardiomyopathy.** Hypertrophy that similarly affects the interventricular septum and left ventricular wall is described as symmetric. On this short-axis left ventricular view there is symmetric hypertrophy of the wall and septum, as well as a prominent and possibly hypertrophied papillary muscles.

Video 7.16

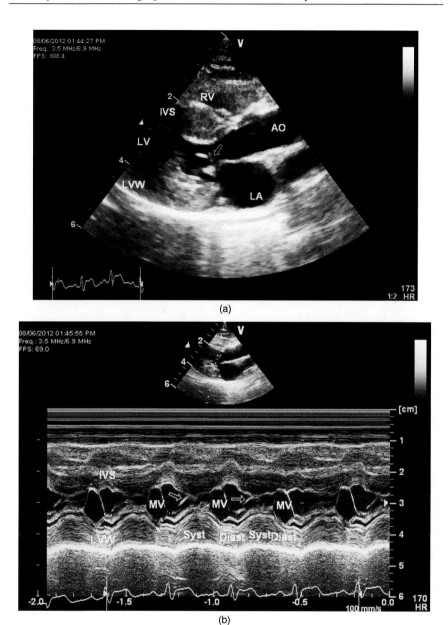

(a)

(b)

Figure 7.17 Hypertrophic cardiomyopathy. (a–d) (a; with Video 7.17) Systolic anterior mitral valve motion (SAM) (arrow) is seen on this long-axis inflow outflow view. This motion of the valve creates an obstruction to left ventricular outflow; (b) SAM (arrows) is seen during systole on this mitral valve M-mode. The M-mode cursor is placed at the tips of the mitral valve leaflets, but may need to be moved into the outflow tract slightly in some cats to display this motion; (c) SAM on this M-mode of the mitral valve has anterior motion for almost all of systole consistent with more significant obstruction than that seen in panel (b); (d) The dynamic nature of outflow obstruction in hypertrophic cardiomyopathy is seen on this M-mode image of the mitral valve. The arrow points at SAM, which is not seen during the next two systolic time periods but is seen again on the last systolic time period.

Video 7.17

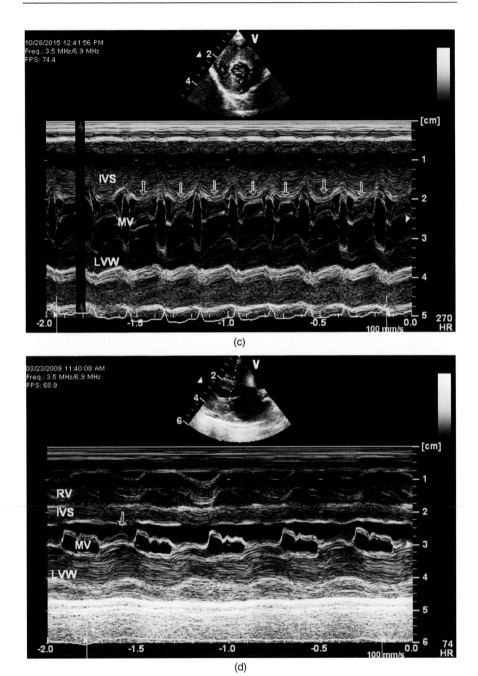

(c)

(d)

Figure 7.17 (*Continued*)

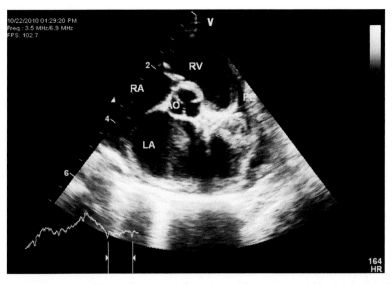

Figure 7.18 Hypertrophic cardiomyopathy. The swirling echoes within this large left atrium represents "smoke" which is highly likely to form thrombus. There is also a thrombus (arrow) in the tip of the left atrial appendage.

Video 7.18

- Thrombus or "smoke" (also called spontaneous echo contrast) is possible within the left atrium and auricle (see Figure and Video 7.18)
- Pleural and pericardial effusions are occasionally seen (see Figure and Video 7.19)

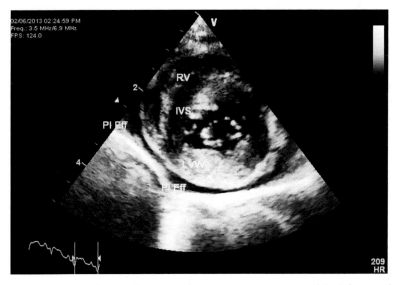

Figure 7.19 Hypertrophic cardiomyopathy. This transverse image of the left ventricle shows hypertrophic walls and a small amount of pleural effusion surrounding the heart. Pleural effusion typically has an irregular border compared to pericardial effusion, which is usually evenly distributed around the heart.

Video 7.19

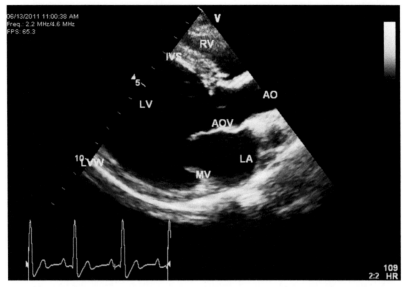

Figure 7.20 Dilated cardiomyopathy. There is significant left ventricular dilation and a mildly dilated left atrium in this heart. The walls are thin relative to the chamber size. The mitral valve appears to be thickened on the video during systole when chordae tendineae are prominent, but the leaflets appear thin and normal during diastole. There is reduced motion of the mitral valve towards the septum, reflecting the large EPSS (mitral valve E point to septal separation). There is clearly reduced function.

Video 7.20

Dilated Cardiomyopathy

- Features
  - Dilated left ventricle (see Figures and Videos 7.20–7.21)
    - Dilation not always present or may be minimal
  - Dilated left atrium (see Figures and Videos 7.20–7.21)
  - Thrombus is possible in the atrium, auricle, or ventricle (rare in dogs)
  - Poor fractional shortening (see Figures 7.20–7.24 and Videos 7.20–7.22)
    - Large left ventricular systolic dimension
    - Reduced fractional shortening and a large systolic dimension occurs before dilation
  - Normal to thin wall and septum
  - Increased E peak to septal separation (EPSS) (see Figure 7.25 and Videos 7.20 and 7.21)
  - Other findings may include pericardial or pleural effusions (see Figures and Videos 7.21–7.22)

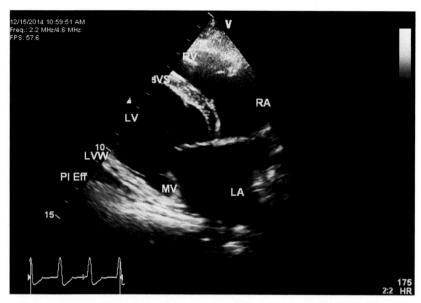

Figure 7.21 Dilated cardiomyopathy. Left ventricular and left atrial dilation is visible on this right parasternal four-chamber. Right ventricular dilation and perhaps right atrial dilation is also present. Mitral valve motion is reduced (large E point to septal separation). There is obvious reduced right and left ventricular systolic function on the video. A small amount of pleural effusion is seen below the left ventricular wall.

Video 7.21

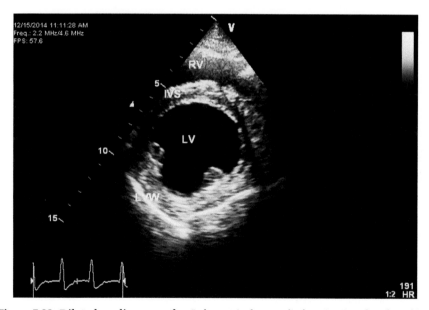

Figure 7.22 Dilated cardiomyopathy. Left ventricular systolic function is reduced on this right parasternal transverse view of the left ventricle. There is a small pleural effusion below the left ventricular wall visible on the video.

Video 7.22

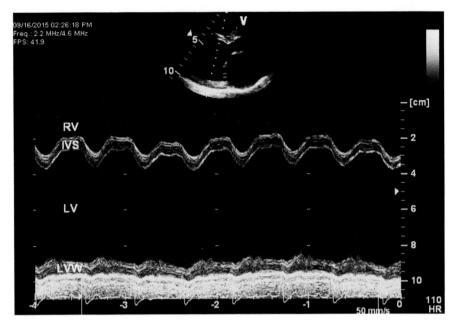

Figure 7.23 Dilated cardiomyopathy. This left ventricular M-mode shows reduced fractional shortening. The left ventricular systolic chamber size is large for a dog of this size. Often, the interventricular septum exhibits more motion than the left ventricular wall.

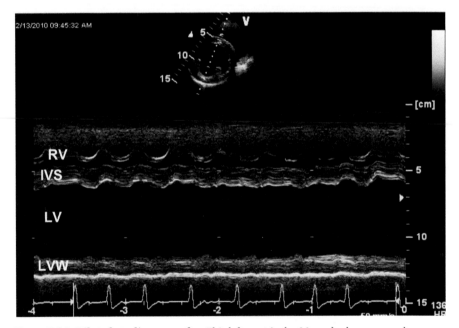

Figure 7.24 Dilated cardiomyopathy. This left ventricular M-mode shows severely reduced contractility. The left ventricular systolic chamber size is large and the fractional shortening is extremely poor. There is very little wall or septal motion.

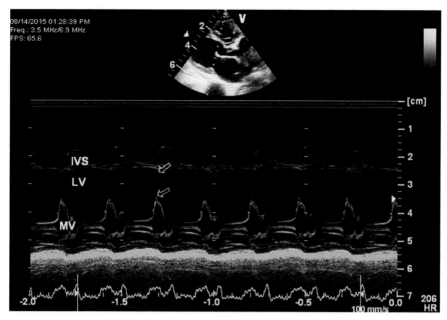

Figure 7.25 Dilated cardiomyopathy. Upward mitral valve motion is reduced in dilated cardiomyopathy because of the reduced volume moving through the valve into the left ventricular chamber. The result is a large EPSS (distance between arrows).

Unclassified Cardiomyopathy

- Features (see Figures and Videos 7.26–7.29)
  - Normal to mildly dilated left ventricle
  - Normal to mildly hypertrophied or thin areas of wall and septum
    - Irregular endocardial surface possible
    - Fibrosis within the myocardium and endocardium (bright echogenic areas) possible
    - Areas of infarction (lack of visible myocardium)
  - Dilated left atrium – always present
    - Thrombus or smoke within the left atrium and auricle is common
  - Possible right atrial dilation
  - Normal to mildly depressed fractional shortening

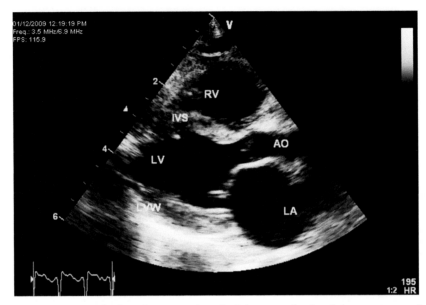

Figure 7.26 Unclassified cardiomyopathy. The left ventricular chamber may appear to be perfectly normal in unclassified cardiomyopathy, as seen on the right parasternal inflow outflow view of the heart in this cat. The left atrial size is large, however, a hallmark feature of this disease. The right ventricle also appears large in this cat.

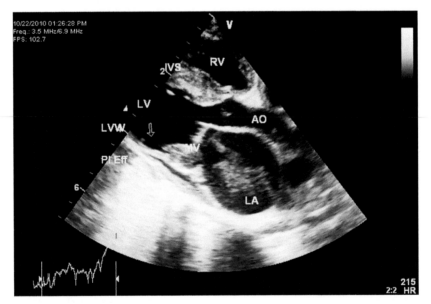

Figure 7.27 Unclassified cardiomyopathy. This right parasternal inflow outflow view shows irregularities in myocardial thickness, the absence of myocardium in one area (arrow) representing infarcted muscle, a large left atrium with "smoke," reduced left ventricular systolic function, and pericardial and plural effusions. The right ventricle appears normal.

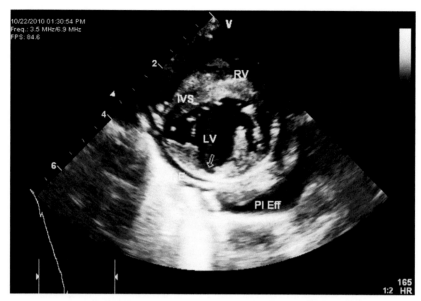

Figure 7.28 Unclassified cardiomyopathy. The left ventricular myocardium shows irregularities in thickness, with a lack of myocardium between the papillary muscles on the left ventricular wall representing infarcted muscle, reduced systolic function, and pleural and pericardial effusions.

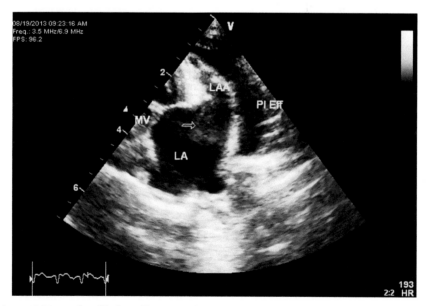

Figure 7.29 Unclassified cardiomyopathy. Smoke (arrow) is seen within this large left atrial and auricular chamber on a left parasternal cranial transverse plane.

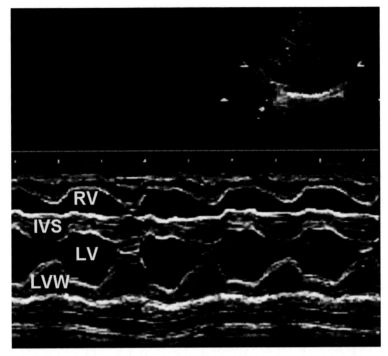

Figure 7.30 Unclassified cardiomyopathy. Left ventricular chamber size, wall thicknesses and systolic function may be normal in hearts with unclassified cardiomyopathy, as is seen here. Despite this, these hearts have large left atriums that reveal the significant heart disease and diastolic dysfunction present in unclassified cardiomyopathy.

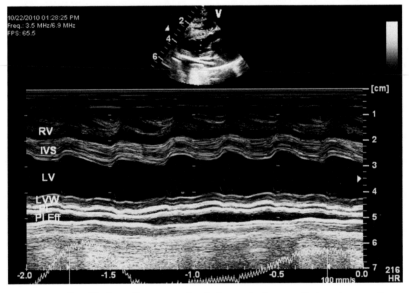

Figure 7.31 Unclassified cardiomyopathy. Left ventricular systolic function may be poor in cats with unclassified cardiomyopathy, especially if areas of the myocardium are infarcted, as is seen in this M-mode's left ventricular wall.

Pericardial Effusion

- Features (see Figures 7.32–7.34)
    - ○ Fluid around the heart appears as a black space
    - ○ Fluid generally is not present much beyond the junction of the atrium and ventricle
    - ○ Fluid space takes the shape of the heart with a smooth border for the peri-cardial sac
        - ■ An irregular shape to the fluid is usually consistent with pleural fluid
    - ○ Pericardial tamponade may be present
        - ■ Right atrial and ventricular wall collapse (see Figure 7.32)
        - ■ Does not have to be a massive effusion
    - ○ Searching for masses is easiest when fluid is present
        - ■ Many masses are missed after fluid is tapped from the sac

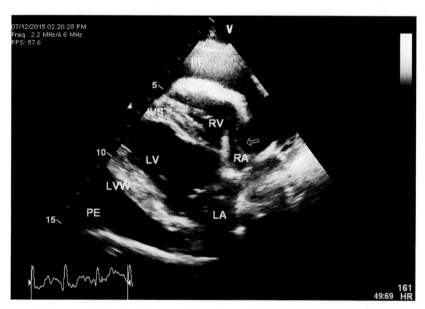

Figure 7.32 Pericardial effusion. Pericardial effusion is a black fluid space with a pericardial sac that usually has a smooth border around the ventricular chambers. Fluid does not extend around the top of heart base. In this right parasternal four-chamber view there is also tamponade (arrow): collapse of the right atrial wall because intrapericardial pressure is higher than right atrial pressure.

Video 7.32

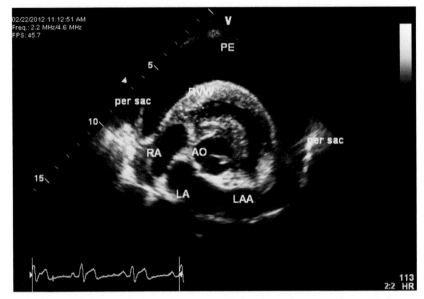

Figure 7.33 Pericardial effusion. This right parasternal transverse heart base shows pericardial effusion around the right ventricular chamber, but not the heart base.

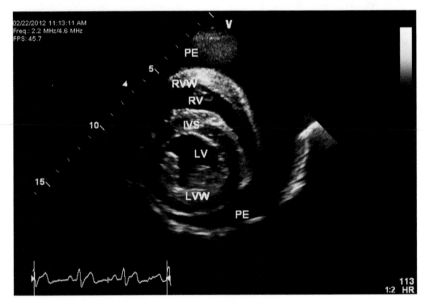

Figure 7.34 Pericardial effusion. This transverse view of the left ventricle shows a black fluid-filled pericardial sac. The fluid takes the shape of the heart and the interior surface of the pericardial sac is smooth.

Hemangiosarcoma

- Features (see Figures and Videos 7.35–7.38)
  - ○ Pericardial effusion if the tumor has bled into the sac
  - ○ Mass seen most commonly at the right atrial appendage
    - ■ Best seen from left-sided cranial long-axis view of the right auricle
  - ○ Masses may be seen anywhere in the right ventricular wall or right atrium, however
  - ○ They are uncommonly seen within the left side of the heart
  - ○ Masses seen outside the right auricle on left-sided views may be aortic body tumors or hemangiosarcoma. Use other views to help differentiate
  - ○ Without effusion many masses are missed
  - ○ Stand the animal up and image it on both sides while it is standing, as the heart shifts in the fluid and different vantages are seen

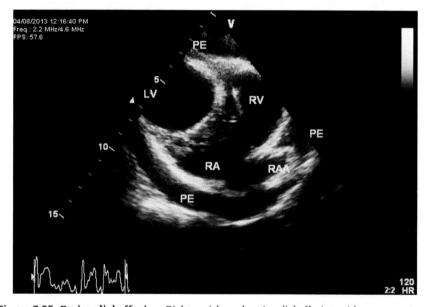

Figure 7.35 Pericardial effusion. Right auricle and pericardial effusion without a mass on this left parasternal cranial long axis plane.

Video 7.35

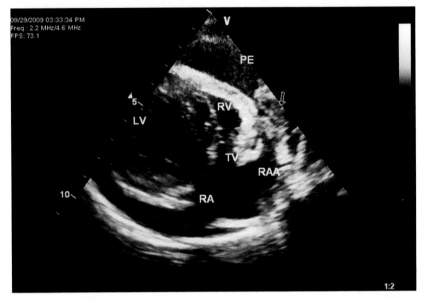

Figure 7.36 Hemangiosarcoma. This left cranial long-axis view of the right atrium and auricle shows a mass on the tip of the atrial appendage (arrow). The mass is easily seen because it is surrounded by pericardial fluid. Without the effusion this mass may be missed.

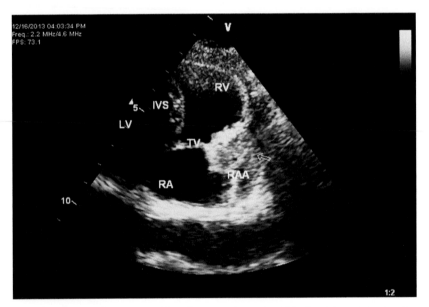

Figure 7.37 Hemangiosarcoma. There is a mass (arrow) within the right atrial appendage on this left cranial long-axis view of the right atrium and auricle. There is no pericardial effusion here. The mass is seen because it is within the chamber.

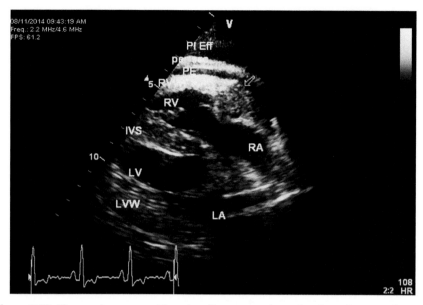

Figure 7.38 Hemangiosarcoma. There is a discrete mass located at the atrioventricular junction (arrow) on this right parasternal four-chamber view. The fibrinous irregularities on seen the outside of the pericardial sac in the video are an expected finding with pleural effusion.

Video 7.38

Aortic Body Tumors

- Features (see Figures and Videos 7.39–7.40)
  - ○ Often no effusion
  - ○ Masses always associated with the aorta
    - On right or left parasternal transverse views
      - □ seen between the right and left atrium
      - □ seen between aorta and pulmonary artery and at the pulmonary artery bifurcation
  - ○ Masses seen outside the right auricle on left-sided views may be aortic body tumors or hemangiosarcoma. Use other views to help differentiate
  - ○ Large masses may compress or invade the atria or great vessels, causing heart failure
    - It is difficult to assess whether they are in or out of the chambers – color flow Doppler is helpful

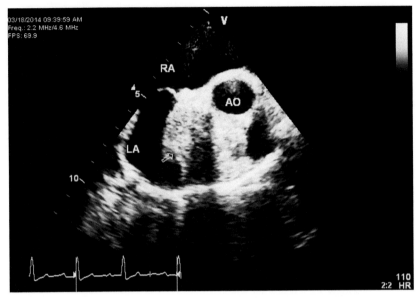

Figure 7.39 Chemodectoma. These lesions (arrow) are typically homogeneous in appearance and associated with the aorta, as seen on this right parasternal transverse view of the heart base. The shadow through the middle of this mass is not a hypoechoic section of the mass, but a refractive shadow from the aorta.

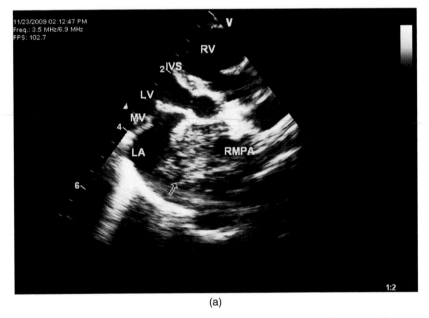

(a)

Figure 7.40 Chemodectoma. (a) Heart base tumors can become very large (see also Video 7.40a). A large homogenous mass is seen associated with the aorta (arrow) on the long axis inflow outflow view; (b) The same mass (arrows) is seen on transverse heart base images (see also Video 7.40b). It is seen associated with the aorta and around the bifurcation of the pulmonary artery.

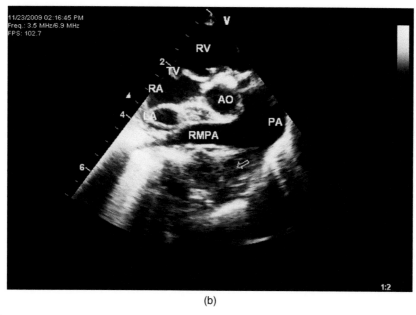

(b)

Figure 7.40 (*Continued*)

Endocarditis

- Features (see Figures and Videos 7.41–7.43)
  - ○ Valvular lesions
    - ■ Small to medium lesions cannot be differentiated from degenerative lesions if on the mitral valve
    - ■ Large irregular lesions are highly suspicious of endocarditis – but this is a clinical diagnosis
    - ■ Aortic valve irregularities should always be suspect for endocarditis
    - ■ They are usually dense and bright in appearance
    - ■ They may be undulating and prolapsing
  - ○ Left ventricular dilation
    - ■ Severity is dependent on the degree of mitral or aortic regurgitation

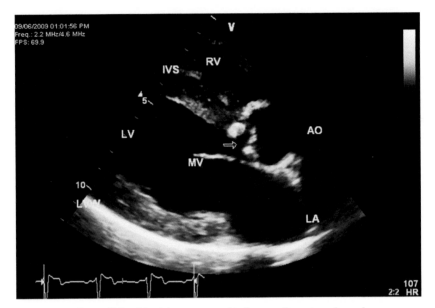

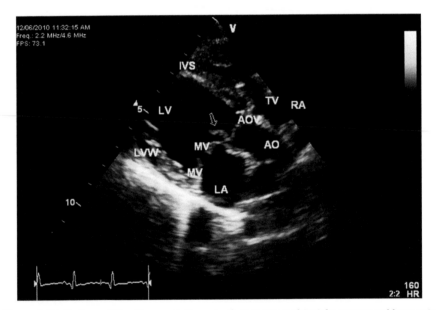

Figure 7.41 **Endocarditis.** This right parasternal inflow outflow view shows large hyperechoic lesions (arrow) associated with the aortic valve. These hyperechoic lesions are typical of endocarditis. The left ventricular chamber is mildly dilated.

Video 7.41

Figure 7.42 **Endocarditis.** The vegetative growth (arrow) on this right parasternal long-axis view of the heart is isoechoic with the aortic and mitral valve leaflets, and wispy in nature.

Video 7.42

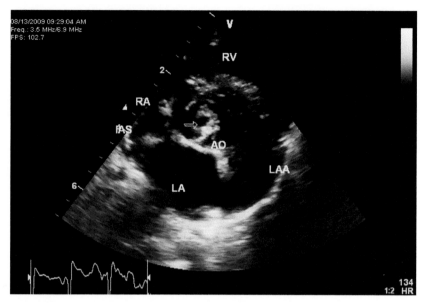

Figure 7.43 Endocarditis. This right parasternal transverse view of the heart base shows vegetative growth associated with the three aortic valve cusps.

Video 7.43

Recommended Reading

The list below consists mostly of textbooks that provide a good base of knowledge for endeavors into the field of echocardiography, its techniques, and its diagnostics. These will enhance your understanding of cardiac ultrasound and cardiac diseases.

1 Berne, R.M. and Levy, M.N. (2001) *Cardiovascular Physiology*, 8th edition. Mosby, St Louis, MO.
2 Boon, J.A. (2011) *Veterinary Echocardiography*, 2nd edition, Wiley Blackwell, Philadelphia, PA.
3 Darke, P., Bonagura, J.D., and Kelly, D.F. (1996) *Color Atlas of Veterinary Cardiology*. Mosby-Wolfe, London, England.
4 Gordon, S.G. and Estrada, A.H. (2013) *The ABCDs of Small Animal Cardiology*. LifeLearn, Guelph, Canada.
5 Braunwald, E., Zipes, D.P., and Libby, P. (eds) (2001) *Heart Disease*, 6th edition. W.B. Saunders Company, Philadelphia, PA.
6 *Kirk's Current Veterinary Therapy XII* (1995) Small Animal Practice. Section 9: Cardiopulmonary Disorders (ed. J.D. Bonagura), W.B. Saunders Company, Philadelphia, PA, pp. 773–930.
7 *Kirk's Current Veterinary Therapy XV* (2014) Small Animal Practice (ed. J.D. Bonagura), Elsevier, St Loius, Missouri.
8 Kittleson, M.D. and Kienle, R.D. (1998) *Small Animal Cardiovascular Medicine*. Mosby, St Louis, MO.
9 Kittleson, M.D. (1994) Left ventricular function and failure. *Part I. Comp. Small Anim.*, **16**, 287–308.
10 Kittleson, M.D. (1994) Left ventricular function and failure. *Part II. Comp. Small Anim.*, **16**, 1001–1017.
11 Tilley, L.P. and Goodwin, J.K. (eds) (2001) *Manual of Canine and Feline Cardiology*, 3rd edition. W.B. Saunders Company, Philadelphia, PA.
12 Weyman, A.E. (ed.) (1994) *Principles and Practice of Echocardiography*, 2nd edition. Lea & Febiger, Philadelphia, PA.
13 Thomas, W.P., Gaber, C.E., Jacobs, G.J., *et al.* (1993) Recommendations for standards in transthoracic two-dimensional echocardiography in the dog and cat. *J. Vet. Intern. Med.*, **7**, 247–252.

Two-Dimensional and M-Mode Echocardiography for the Small Animal Practitioner, Second Edition. June A. Boon.
© 2017 John Wiley & Sons, Inc. Published 2017 by John Wiley & Sons, Inc.
Companion Website: www.wiley.com/go/boon/two-dimensional

Glossary

AMV	anterior mitral valve leaflet
AMV	anterior mitral valve
Ant AO wall	anterior aortic wall
AO	aorta
Ao	aorta
AOV	aortic valve
CA VC	caudal vena cava
CI	confidence interval
CR VC	cranial vena cava
CT	chordae tendineae
d	diastole
dias	diastole
diast	diastole
IAS	interatrial septum
IVS	interventricular septum
LA	left atrium
LAA	left atrial appendage
LC	left coronary cusp of the aortic valve
LMPA	left main pulmonary artery
LV	left ventricle
LVW	left ventricular wall
mm	millimeter
MV	mitral valve
MV A	mitral valve A peak
MV AL	mitral valve anterior leaflet
MV E	mitral valve E peak
MV PL	mitral valve posterior leaflet
NC	noncoronary cusp of the aortic valve
PA	pulmonary artery
PE	pericardial effusion

Two-Dimensional and M-Mode Echocardiography for the Small Animal Practitioner, Second Edition. June A. Boon.
© 2017 John Wiley & Sons, Inc. Published 2017 by John Wiley & Sons, Inc.
Companion Website: www.wiley.com/go/boon/two-dimensional

per sac	pericardial sac
Pl Eff	pleural effusion
PM	papillary muscle
PMV	posterior mitral valve
Post AO wall	posterior aortic wall
PV	pulmonary valve
RA	right atrium
RAA	right atrial appendage
RC	right coronary cusp of the aortic valve
RMPA	right main pulmonary artery
RV	right ventricle
RVW	right ventricular wall
sys	systole
syst	systole
Syst	systole
TV	tricuspid valve
VC	vena cava (caudal)

Index

afterload   92, 94
anatomy, cardiac   2
aorta
   apical five-chamber view   50
   left cranial transverse view   46
   measurements   86–89
   M-mode imaging   78–80
   reference values   95–103
   right parasternal heart base views   39–42
   right parasternal inflow outflow view   26, 28, 29
aortic body tumors   133–135
aortic valve   43
   endocarditis   135–137
A peak, mitral valve   81, 82
apical five-chamber view   50, 73–74
apical four-chamber view   49, 69–73
applications, echocardiography   1

cardiomyopathy
   dilated   122–125
   hypertrophic   29, 30, 92, 116–121
   unclassified   125–128
cats
   apical four-chamber view   72–73
   four-chamber view   32
   left auricle view   47–48, 69
   left ventricular inflow outflow view   29–31, 55–56
   orientation of heart in thorax   4
   reference values   95
chemodectoma   134–135
chordae tendineae
   right parasternal transverse view   38–39
   ruptured   108, 111
compounding   23
contractility   91, 92, 94
   degenerative mitral valve disease   112, 114
   dilated cardiomyopathy   124
cross beam   23

degenerative mitral valve disease   108–116
depth, adjusting   7–8

dilated cardiomyopathy   122–125
dogs
   apical four-chamber view   69–72
   four-chamber view   31–32, 33–34, 35
   left ventricular inflow outflow view   25–29, 52–55
   orientation of heart in thorax   3
   reference values   96–103
dynamic range   15–16

endocarditis   135–137
E peak, mitral valve   80–82
E peak to septal separation (EPSS)   89–90, 103
   dilated cardiomyopathy   122, 123, 125

focus   18–19
four-chamber view   31–35
   scanning technique   56–59
fractional shortening   91, 93–94
   degenerative mitral valve disease   112, 114
   dilated cardiomyopathy   122, 124
   reference values   95–103
frequency, transducer   8–10

gain   10–11
grey map   14–15

hair removal   4–5
harmonics   20–21
heart
   anatomy   2
   orientation in thorax   3–4
heart base
   left cranial transverse views   45–48, 67–69
   right parasternal transverse views   39–42, 62–64
heart rate (HR)   103
hemangiosarcoma   131–133
hypertrophic (obstructive) cardiomyopathy   29, 30, 92, 116–121

image quality, improving   7–23
imaging planes, two-dimensional   24–50

Two-Dimensional and M-Mode Echocardiography for the Small Animal Practitioner, Second Edition. June A. Boon.
Companion Website: www.wiley.com/go/boon/two-dimensional